Sickle Cell Disease
100 Years Later

By Dan Moore, Sr. &
Phyllis Zachery-Thomas

ISBN 1453603824 EAN-13 9781453603826.

All proceeds from the book support
Marrow For Life, Inc., SCD Soldier Network, Inc.
and the FACE Foundation, Inc.

Dedicated To
All the patients, families, organizations,
health care providers, researchers and friends
associated with sickle cell, its prevention, treatment
and its cure.

Special Thanks To
Ariel Howard, Michele Mitchell, Elena Moore,
Estella Moore, Asia Rahman and Joyce Washington
for their invaluable contributions and the "Be The Match"
Team, Tina, Rod and Stacy and The APEX Museum in
Atlanta for its tireless efforts and support of Marrow For
Life.

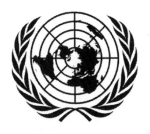

United Nations
World Sickle Cell Day
June 19

United Nations Resolution A/63/L63 recognizes sickle cell disease as a public health problem. This resolution, which was initiated by the Paris-based International Organization for the fight against Sickle Cell Disease (OILD/SCDIO), was proposed by a delegation from the Republic of Congo Brazzaville and co-sponsored by 24 Member States. Among the objectives of this resolution was in particular the celebration on June 19th of each year, a World Day of Sickle Cell Disease devoted to awareness campaigns at national and international levels.

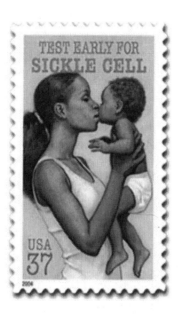

In 2004 the Sickle Cell Disease Awareness Stamp was created raising public awareness of health and social issues. The inscription "Test Early for Sickle Cell" conveys the importance of early testing.

Introduction

Although this country is reaching the 100 year landmark of the discovery of sickle cell disease, it has been a battle waged by people of African descent for centuries. We have covered much ground as a nation, but the terrain is vast and there is more to be explored. The major problem faced in the 21st century by those who suffer from this debilitating disease is lack of awareness. Today, the only known cure for sickle cell is a bone marrow, stem cell or umbilical cord transplant, and the chances for finding a matching donor within the national registry are slim-to-none for African Americans. This dilemma exists because there are not enough African Americans on the registry to help other African Americans in need.

I know that if the Black community were aware of the suffering experienced by children and adults with sickle cell, they would race to the nearest center to join the registry. The stories you are about to read are the personal testimonies of survivors. This book was created in order to bring the human connection to those in need, and those who can help. At present, there is a gap within the Black community that must be filled. Our destiny is in our hands and we must rise to the challenge placed at our feet and close this gap. The gap is awareness. Many of us do not know that we can save someone's life today. We do not know that we can end a child's 'pain crisis.' We can prevent another stroke. We can be the reason that an African American lives.

It is my hope that these stories will help to close the gap that exists and drive more African Americans to join the National Marrow Donor "Be The Match Registry" so future generations of African-Americans will not have to tell the same stories you will read within these pages.

Michele Mitchell
Chief Researcher, Marrow For Life
PhD candidate

Table of Contents

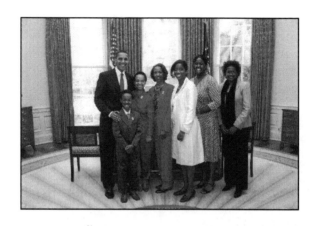

President Barack Obama meets with
Sickle Cell Disease Association of America.

Sickle Cell Soldiers

The Story of A SCD Soldier

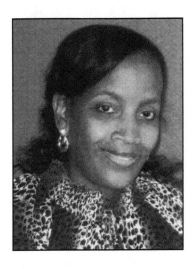

Phyllis Zachery-Thomas

As far back as I can remember, I knew that I had sickle cell anemia. I was diagnosed when I was six months old, and still my father and mother had no idea what that diagnosis meant. They are both deceased now, so many of my questions will forever go unanswered. I have questions like, "Why did you go on to have two more children after I was born? Did you understand the odds of having another baby with the disease?" I would venture to bet that they were totally unaware of what took place. Why am I so sure about that? It's because in 2010 we are celebrating 100 years, since the first case of sickle cell was described in western literature and many people still don't have a clue as to what the disease is. I don't want to get caught up in telling you all about the blood disorder, and neglect to tell you the most important thing – how I have dealt with the effects of it.

As a child, I was very sick and was in and out of the hospital quite often. My mother received so many predictions about my life expectancy that I know that God had to strengthen her. I remember that there was some talk about me not reaching the age of 13, and after I did, the next prediction was age 21 then 30. Oh well, so much for statistics. I just kept right on living. Don't get me wrong, it wasn't an easy life by any means. Although I was born in Dallas, TX, and returned there as a teenager, my family moved to Los Angeles when I was approximately five years old. We lived there for about 10 years, so, in many regards, I consider myself a native of Los Angeles because I spent my formative years there. I lived right in the middle of what is now known as South Central at 6605 Victoria. It's amazing the things that you remember.

My hospital was Daniel Freeman in Inglewood, CA and I loved my doctor and the nurses who cared for me. My mother was my constant companion whenever I was hospitalized and I often wonder how difficult that must have been, considering she had four children. My oldest brother was oftentimes with the Garcia family down the street; so he was in good hands. My younger brother is only two years younger than I am and he was the one child she couldn't leave with anyone. He always tagged along, so

I think of all of my siblings, he has a better understanding of my battle with sickle cell. Then there was my baby sister, she ended up spending time away from us, because it was just too much on my mother after she and my father separated. My mom sent her to my grandmother for a short amount of time, until she was able to work out a plan.

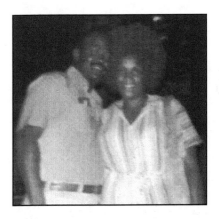

My father & mother

I was in and out of the hospital so often. Then something happened that makes me shake my head to this day. Neither my mom nor I knew it at the time, but there was another little girl who was about three years younger than me who also had sickle cell anemia, and a lot of times, she was in the hospital at the same time as me. She looked so much like me that the staff would call her by my name and we even shared the same last name. One of my nurses brought this to the attention of our doctors and suggested that one of us be moved to another hospital, because she suspected that we were sisters and our mothers were not aware of each other. It turns out that she was right. My stepsister could not have been more like me if she had been my twin. It wasn't until I was an adult that I actually met her, but not only did we look alike, write alike and enjoy sunflower seeds, we apparently had the same triggers. Triggers are things that lead you into a pain crisis, like cold weather, stress, infections, etc. Whenever I was in a pain crisis, chances were that so was she. I can't believe that we didn't bump into each other at the hospital; it would have been like a scene right out of a movie. She later told me that she knew she had other siblings but didn't know their names. Her encounter with my father was brief. Although he did marry her mom, I think that they separated shortly after her birth. My dad returned to my mother and had my baby sister about three years after my stepsister was born. In any case, we were glad to have the chance to know one another. Somehow my mom received word that my father had a daughter who wanted to meet us. My mom facilitated the meeting by talking with my stepsister's mom and exchanging contact information. We ended up forming a real sisterly bond and I was so happy to have her in my life. I was already an adult and living in Dallas, TX with my husband and daughter. My stepsister was in Los Angeles, so I sent for her. She came to Dallas and spent the entire summer with me. She had a chance to meet my father's side of the family and get to know her other brothers and sisters. She looked so much like us it was an instant acceptance, which helped her fill in some of the gaps in her life. Unfortunately she lost her battle with sickle cell disease in June of 2006.

My stepsister's name was Kimberly Dana Zachery and like many with sickle cell disease, she was in constant battle with the blood disorder that threatened her quality of life. When she was well, she was able to work as a beautician and she had an infectious personality. Kim loved life and she loved family. I knew that she was my sister when I first saw her picture, received her first letter and heard her voice over the phone. When she died, I went to Los Angeles to pay my final respect, but what happened to me that day changed the entire course of my life.

It was not until this very moment that I now know what led me down the road to forming SCD Soldier Network, Inc. I thought that writing my story would be too much. I didn't know exactly what I would say. Right here and right now I know where the story begins. It begins with me looking into Kim's casket and seeing myself, coming face to face with my own mortality.

Kimberly Dana Zachery

The Story Before the Story

How Sickle Cell Wreaked Havoc on My Life

Let's rewind for just a minute because the summer that I met Kim, I was in a very good place. I was never sick, I was working in the accounting department of a bank and I loved the hand that life dealt to me. As a matter of fact, for nearly ten years it was as if I didn't even have sickle cell. I was in ministry at my church and I had an incredible testimony of how God had healed me from the disease that taunted me my entire childhood. I wanted that for Kim so much, that I may have completely turned her off. I was what they call a "hot mess." I was a hot gospel mess, because I had no room for sickness in my testimony. It was a thing of the past and my relationship with God was solid as a rock. You don't realize how arrogant you can be when your life is going so well, until it stops and like Job of the Bible, all hell breaks loose on you. It will make you take a serious look at yourself and everything around you.

After experiencing good health, all of a sudden, I began to have the fight of my life. Sickle Cell waged its war on me and threatened everything that was not built on a solid foundation. I was in and out of the hospital so much that I began to like the food there and it became my second home. Everyone knew the drill from the ER department to food service. I ordered from the special meal menu for those with extended stays and the tray passers would make sure I had my favorite foods available from the kitchen. The nurses even began to know me intimately. They were able to chart the development of my daughter, and for the first time in my adult life, I was beginning to be ok with meeting other adults with sickle cell disease. I had been so disconnected from the sickle cell community and the idea of relying on a support group was going to take a miracle. I had no desire to get that close, but I was at least open to meeting others who were in the hospital at the same time that I was.

Alone & Isolated

I was now in a very lonely place spiritually, because although I was getting a sense of what was going on in my life, the people at church weren't. My testimony was so powerful that I don't think anyone was willing to hear anything that did not support the confession that I was healed. I heard everything from "the devil is trying to steal your testimony" to "the devil is a lie." The devil is a liar, but he wasn't lying about the pain I was experiencing. It was very much the truth. I couldn't convince anyone that my suffering was going to serve a much bigger purpose than my healing ever did. I was the only one who believed that. Even though I believed it with every ounce of faith that I possessed, I couldn't explain how. My mother tried to understand it, but as an onlooker she was torn because she couldn't see the necessity of so much pain. My pastor was not going to assist me in accepting what had happened as the will of God. He wanted this to just be a test and not the end to the healing that I was so proud to testify of. In a lot of ways I think that they all thought I lost my faith somewhere down the line, but I hadn't. I knew that my season for health was over and I didn't know if it would ever return. All I had to count on was that God had not abandoned me and that He was in total control of this situation. It seems so easy to explain now, but back then I just wanted people to know that I was in good hands. I have a cousin who spent many nights with me in the hospital and was a witness to my late night battles with the pain. She, at some point, asked God to give her my pain. His answer to her was "Every man has his own cross to bear". I understood that and I just wanted to be left alone to deal with what was happening. I respected the relationship that I had with those individuals who I was in ministry with, but I didn't know how to ignore their desire for me to be healed, while listening to God who was saying "My grace is sufficient". I eventually left the church that I adored in exchange for TV and radio ministry. I still needed to be fed spiritually, but more than anything I needed a word from God that helped me to bring glory to His name through my pain. I needed God to talk to me, I needed Him to comfort me and explain what was happening to me. I was becoming ashamed of the battle that I was in. Why was I identifying with Job? Why is everybody asking why this is happening instead of helping me to get through it? I hadn't committed some God-awful sin. I was a little arrogant and perhaps I had my father on a pedestal that belonged to God, but was I being punished for that? I needed answers and only God could provide them for me. I wasn't being punished but God revealed something to me that broke my heart. He showed me that I had allowed Him into every area of my life, except the 'Daddy Zone'. That was my sacred little place and not even God could go there. My daddy was on the throne and could not be removed. I was determined to see him through rose-colored glasses and as a result of that decision I was doomed to keep his bloodline. God had offered me a better father-daughter relationship and I neglected to accept it. You don't have to be super spiritual to understand this. God had become my Protector, Provider, Husband and Healer, but He did not make the father position in my life. Only God could have revealed that to me. At one point, my pastor was right on target as he began to bring up my father. He wanted me to explore my relationship with my dad, but I didn't quite get where he was coming from so it wasn't received well. I don't think anyone could have gotten me to see that because I was in so much denial. But now when I say I'm a King's Kid I mean it. God is truly my father and if I never experience another day of healing, it is ok with me, because opening myself and allowing God to be my everything was worth the price I had to pay.

Sickle Cell Effected Every Thing in My Life

It wasn't long before my husband grew lonely and turned to his buddies and alcohol as a distraction to what was happening to us. Later he exchanged his buddies for women. This disease was determined to rip my life into shreds. It was going to cause a huge wedge between my church and I, it caused my daughters to be alone without parental guidance and people on the outside knew very little about what was going on. The battle with sickle cell was affecting the entire family and because it was so devastating it created a deafening silence. I really feel that my husband was ill equipped to handle this and no one saw that he was sinking except women who were more than happy to soothe his broken heart. It's not like I think that other woman were to blame for my husband's infidelity because he had an obligation to abide by the commitment that he vowed to uphold. Cheating is a subject that will always spark great debates and people disagree when it comes to whether or not someone can make you cheat, but I can honestly say that I had a lot to do with the isolation that he felt. Before you begin to judge our situation, let me paint the picture of the life that we had together.

I met Phillip over the phone when I was a teenager. He went to school with two of my cousins and we were introduced during one of my stays in the hospital. I was still in high school at the time and I was always on the phone whenever I had to be in the hospital. This particular day I was talking with my cousin when Phillip called her house looking for her brother. She told him that she was on the phone with me and he wanted in on the conversation. I believe she clicked us in on a three-way call and introduced us to each other. We talked a couple of times while I was in the hospital and a few more times prior to meeting face to face. I not only battled sickle cell anemia, I also had lupus and was on medication that had me very swollen. I was not feeling very good about my appearance, but being young I was bold enough to meet a stranger in hopes that he would like what he saw. To this day I don't really know how he felt when he saw me, but he made me feel like a million dollar bill. We met at the Fair Park of Texas in the midway, which is where the amusement park rides are. It wasn't fair season, but they would open the midway during the summer. When I saw him I was a little torn and didn't know if I really liked him, but he grabbed my hand and we walked up and down the midway strip. The thing that really won me over was the fact that he was so popular. Every other person that we ran into knew him and whenever he stopped to speak, he held my hand tighter and pulled me in closer. That made a major impact on me because it was a vast difference from my past boyfriend. He didn't like the fact that I had gained so much weight from the medication, but Phillip didn't seem to mind. He made me feel like I was beautiful. We didn't stay together very long before I backed away from the relationship because of my own self esteem issues. I went on to graduate high school and Phillip went into the military. As soon as he got out of basic training he came back looking for me and he found me. I was now ready to be his lady for life.

Phillip and I were married and he landed a full-time job with the Texas National Guard so we could stay together in Dallas, near my doctors and our family. It wasn't long before we had our daughter, Candis. Phillip already had a child when I met him and I was ok with that, because I was young and in love. His daughter was my daughter so when Candis was born I wanted her to know her stepsister Myessha. We were the young family to be. Although we were young, we had a bright future. I was working full-time as a retail clerk and Phillip was off to a great start in his career in the Military. We had big dreams that by the time he was 40 he would retire and I would be able to stop working and we would travel. There wasn't anything I wanted that Phillip wasn't willing to get for me. I felt smothered at times and being young, I thought it was cute to "need my space". Not cute ladies, sometimes you will get more space than you know what to do with. Phillip was always right under me and I encouraged him to have a life beyond me. It didn't matter what I said, Phillip rushed home every day after work and I could set the timer by his promptness. Whenever I was sick, he did his best to care for me, but I was so mean to him. I was also mean to my mother whenever I was sick, but she knew where it was coming from.

I wanted my daddy to care about what was happening to me. Where was he? Did anyone tell him that I was sick and in the hospital? I was mad that they were trying to fill in the gap. I just wanted my dad. The same man that left our family, had another baby with sickle cell and didn't stick around to see what kind of life either one of us would have. Yes, that's the daddy I had on a pedestal, high and lifted up. He was all I wanted, and since I couldn't have him I was angry at the world. Once I began to experience healing I was able to find out what a father's love felt like. God began to teach me the love of a father, through His love for me. He allowed me to be well for a while and He took away all of the cravings that I had for my dad, because the very thing that I wanted when I was sick was what brought me more pain. I don't know why I only wanted my daddy when I was sick and I turned on my mother and husband when all they were trying to do was fill in the gaps from the abandonment that I was feeling. Maybe one day I will know why I was like that, but for now I must deal with the fact that I made everyone miserable when I was sick. My husband endured so much abuse when I wasn't feeling well that I would say we were in an abusive relationship. I can't believe that I just said that. Was I really that bad? If you ask my husband, I wonder what his answer would be. With me not being sick during those years our life was wonderful, but he never forgot all of the abuse he endured from me. Once the pain from the sickle cell returned, I didn't long for my daddy anymore, because God had taken His proper place in my life. Although I still loved my dad, I was no longer in denial, creating this fantasy of the perfect father that never existed. I also stopped being as mean as I used to be, but now I was confused and frustrated.

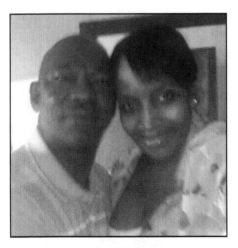

Phillip and me

I was starting to have problems at work because of my attendance and they did not understand, because I had gone so long without any problems. I was always there and I was fully present. They didn't understand that this sudden change was the result of a blood disorder that I had all of my life, because it had not been an issue for me on my job in the past. It came to the point that I had to retire on disability because there was no way that I could keep a job with the frequency of my hospitalizations and the severity of my pain.

No Choice but to Become an Advocate

Becoming my own advocate was mandatory at this point because I had to be able to explain what was going on. I couldn't depend on someone else to do that, because they had no idea how to explain why I hadn't seen a doctor in over seven years when I had a severe form of sickle cell. Most of the people who were in my life at that time knew very little about my previous battle with the disease and were not equipped to assist me. My husband now had to deal with my illness again and because of all of the anger he encountered from my earlier pain episodes he was very distant whenever I was sick. He would stay away and I wanted him near. He couldn't deal with coming home and his wife wasn't there, and he didn't know when I would return. By this time, his daughter Myessha was a teenager and she was living with us and our daughter Candis was a preteen. After about two years my mother suffered a ruptured brain aneurysm and was bed ridden, unable to be the support system that she had been my entire life. My whole life was turned upside down. My husband was not use to having to be the caregiver at home and because the girls were older, he didn't see the problem with leaving them at home alone for long periods of time. His drinking increased and when I was in the hospital he became MIA (missing in action). It was like when I had a sickle cell crisis, he had his own personal crisis. I was at my wits end because I was no longer in church, my family didn't know how to help me, because my mother always did that, and I didn't know how to ask for help. I didn't ask for help mainly because I needed everything, but I didn't know how to express that. Our daughters were building up walls that prevented them from dealing with what was happening and my husband was out on a limb that threatened his very existence.

It seemed that at one point I was in the hospital as much as I was at home. I started meeting people with sickle cell and we formed our own little support group. There are a couple of people that I have to say were instrumental in getting me involved with becoming an advocate for others. First there is TJ, she was this sassy woman who was a ray of sunshine when I met her. She had two children, a daughter who was in college and a son who was in elementary school. There was something about TJ that drew me in.

Me and TJ

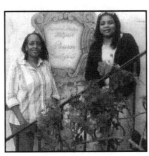

My mother had recently had the aneurysm and it seemed as though her spirit was speaking through TJ. We are in the same age range but she reminded me of my mother so much that it was like an instant bond was created. We had a lot of the same triggers so just like with my sister, whenever I was sick, TJ was probably sick also. She became my new constant companion, my new best friend. I care about her and her kids like they are a part of my family. We would talk every day, two and three times a day. To this day, nobody has ever made that kind of impact on my life. If I started telling you anything more about her and her kids, this book would end up being all about her. I would never be able to finish talking about how special she is to me. If she were having any issues while she was in the hospital I was going to address them for her and if we were in the hospital at the same time, I would encourage her daughter to advocate for her. The second person that I have to mention is Mr. Huguley. He had two daughters and they both became a part of our support group even though only one of them had sickle cell. Galen & Gabby shared their mother and father with us and for me there was something extra special about him and mama Huguley. I felt that he charged me with leading our group and making sure that we always supported one another. I feel like he wasn't in my life long enough, because he was diagnosed with cancer and died with his eyes fixed on me. I will never forget the day that he died. We were at Methodist Hospital in Dallas, TX and Galen was in the room next to her dad and he was in the room at the end of the hall. I was visiting with Galen when the nurse walked in and told us that we needed to come to his room if we wanted to say goodbye because he was on his last few breathes. We helped Galen to gather herself and we walked down the hall together. In my mind it was a very long walk. When we got there Galen took a seat at the head of his bed and began to talk to him. She assured him that she would be ok and that he could go and be with the Lord. I looked into his eyes and it felt as though he was looking to me for confirmation and I nodded yes. Galen then kissed him and he transitioned into the next stage of life. I was devastated and nobody knows how much. I still feel his presence sometimes whenever I am supporting someone through a pain crisis or advocating for them.

My Zest for Life Fades

I wanted to keep our group together, but I was getting tired of all of the breakdowns that were happening around me. My brother and his wife were breaking up, my sister and her husband were breaking up, my mom wasn't getting any better and my husband was straying further away and beginning to have problems on his job. I was sick all of the time, my liver was damaged and I found out that I had a brain aneurysm and although it was tiny, it was there. I was struggling to keep my head above water while battling a blood disease that was creating all sorts of issues that threatened to end my life.

My husband and I separated and I loss my home. My brother and I moved in together and we moved our mother in with us and we became her primary caregivers, although he had already assumed that role from the start. In 2001 my mother passed away and after years of watching her lay in the bed unable to do anything for herself, it was bitter sweet. My mother was so outgoing and never met a stranger. She never waited for people to ask for her help, she met needs as soon as she identified that one existed. We had big hopes that she would recover and it was a constant roller coaster ride. I always felt bad whenever I was in the hospital and couldn't do my part to help with her care. My brother Michael even created a diaper product that made it easy for me to change her whenever I was with her alone. He named it Diaper Mate and he had it patented because it was created in such a way that it was very effective. I know that whenever it makes it to the market place it will help to bring a better quality of care to bed ridden patients.

My Mother's death sucked out the last bit of desire for me to live. My daughter and stepdaughter both lived with me after my brother and I went our separate ways. My daughter graduated the year following my mother's death and I wanted to be alone. My stepdaughter moved to another state and I was hoping that my daughter would get into a local university and live on campus. I was determined to move away and find a peaceful place to die. I told everyone that I was leaving Texas and everyone responded the same way. What about your sickle cell? They wanted to know why I would leave my doctor after finally having a wonderful relationship with her. How was I going to tell them that I didn't care if I had a doctor? I couldn't bring myself to admit out loud that I wanted to die. I started researching cities that had good sickle cell care facilities, just to soothe their minds. I chose Atlanta because of the rave reviews of Grady Hospital's sickle cell program. I had no intention of ever going there. It was just a good answer to give to all of those who were concerned.

My Daughter Candis

My daughter decided that I couldn't go to Atlanta alone so she applied to Georgia State and Clark Atlanta University. We went to Atlanta before she graduated in order to tour the colleges and to look for a place for me to stay. I wanted a small apartment so she would be forced to live on campus. I found the perfect spot not far from the airport but too far from Grady Hospital. I didn't drive much, so my daughter kept the car that her father and I purchased. She was accepted into Clark but because it was a private university it was very expensive. I love my daughter, because she never once expected me to figure out how I would afford for her to go. She contacted the track coach and the volleyball coach in search of a scholarship that would help pay for her college expenses. I couldn't believe that she made it happen when by this time the teams had already been established. She ended up trying out for the volleyball team and received a scholarship. I was so proud of her. It was amazing how she pulled that off just weeks before school was about to start. It was obvious to me that she was operating in the favor of the Lord. Track was really her favorite sport, but I think she was an all around good athlete. I was happy to know that she made the volleyball team. She was good at everything she put her hand to do so it's no wonder that as a freshman in college she made things happen for herself. I hated that it was just the two of us, because it seemed as though I could never make any of her games and I had no one to count on to support her. She was used to that, because I was never very active with her extra-curricular activities when she was in school.

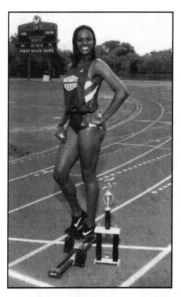

My daughter Candis

I hate that my daughter had to live with the reality of me being unreliable. Not that I didn't want to be there but most of the time I was too sick, tired or depressed to go. Then when I did feel up to it I didn't have transportation or a friend I could count on to take me. Oftentimes I wonder how (living as my daughter) has affected her. She has a very tough exterior and she can't deal with nonsense without overreacting, and at times she seems bitter towards me. Don't get me wrong, I know that she loves me and would trade her life for mine if it were possible. The fact that she wouldn't let me move to Atlanta alone showed me how committed she is to me. Although she lived on campus and had a tight schedule, she always checked on me. I eventually bought a cash car to run my little errands in the neighborhood. I wasn't taking care of myself and she knew it. If she came over and saw that there weren't any groceries, she would ask me for a list and she would make sure that there was plenty food in the house.

When school was out in the summer she landed a job at AirTran Airways working on the ramp. If you knew my daughter, you would be raising your eyebrows because she is so prissy that she just didn't seem like a girl who wanted to work on the ramp. She loved it because it kept her physically active so when it was time to go back to volleyball she would still be in shape. Candis has always commanded the attention of those she came in contact with. When she was in the 7th grade she introduced herself to all of the administrators of her new middle school. The counselor told me how confident and articulate she was. They all thought that she was a teacher's assistant. They could not believe that she was actually a student. She has always carried herself in a way that was much more mature than other kids her age. Because she was tall and well spoken people were always in awe of her, even when she was a toddler. The girl can sing and she loves all sorts of music. She never wanted to pursue it no matter how much we all encouraged it. She did promise to try out for American Idol one year, but that never happened.

If there is anything that I wanted to make sure my daughter understands, it would be that she was the best thing that God has ever given me. With all of our disagreements and moments of discord, I love her like I have never loved anyone. After Candis' second year of college she got pregnant and had my granddaughter Jessica. Now that's my mini me. She was the first thing in a long time that made me want to live. Of course for Candis it was a difficult decision to actually have her because although she and the baby's father were in a good place, she didn't have much faith in the fact that I would be able to help. She is no longer with him, but I will forever be grateful to him for making her discuss her options with me. She knew I would object to anything short of having the baby and keeping it. The day that they called me turned my whole world around. I know that it was probably the hardest call she ever had to make. I promised her that I would do my very best to help with the baby and support her in completing her degree. So when my lease was up I made preparations to move into a larger apartment. It was perfect for the three of us. I gave Candis the biggest room for her and Jessica and I was in heaven. I know that my daughter had to wonder if I could really do all that I promised, but she took a chance and did it anyway.

Things were all ready for Jessica's arrival and within a few months she was born. No matter who they thought she looked like, all I could see was me. She was my muse for living. I was able to keep Jessica while Candis went to school and to work. She was no longer playing volleyball so student loans were her only option. She only made it one semester before dropping out. I was disappointed but I understood. She was a great little mother and although we lived together she took her responsibility for this baby of hers very serious. I had to go into the hospital a couple of times before we came up with a back-up plan. We met a lady who had a home daycare and she kept a few kids whose parents worked crazy hours, which was perfect for us. I was feeling my best although I was hurting everyday from the pain of sickle cell. It was really tough but I was so committed that I kept pushing in spite of the pain.

Soon Candis applied to become a flight attendant. I think she had grown tired of working such a strenuous job. Of course my daughter got the job that I thought she should have had from the beginning. She would be gone days at a time but then she would also be at home days at a time. It was if we were co-parents. Because I didn't drive much, we ended up putting Jessica in a learning center that did pick-ups and drop-offs. So although I would have her days at a time it wasn't like I had to care for her all day. It was a system that worked.

Me and Jessica

Coming to Grips with My Own Mortality

My newfound desire to live that came with Jessica's arrival had begun to fade with each hospitalization. By this time I was taking infusions in my belly for eight hours during the night in order to remove some of the iron overload that I now had. Due to all of the blood transfusions that I have gotten over the years it was taking its toll on me. My liver was damaged and the iron overload needed to be treated right away. I was also having problems with my oxygen supply due to small airway disease. Even now my oxygen level will drop as low as 85% and I won't even know it because I'm use to operating at such a low level. I guess it's just like the low blood counts, I'm used to it. If my hemoglobin drops below a seven I can't necessarily tell because my energy level is always low. The battle of sickle cell disease goes beyond the pain crisis. It's the damaged joints, vital organs that are affected by the lack of oxygen and managing the medications that have serious side effects. I was slowly getting back in the mode of not wanting to fight anymore. I tried so hard to fight those feelings by taking advantage of my travel benefits from my daughter working for the airlines.

My friend TJ was listed as a travel companion on Candis' travel benefits so if I went into the hospital she could just hop on a plane and fill in for me. What kind of friend does that? Although TJ and I are around the same age, I have always felt her motherly touch in my life. It was also good for her because her son was going to be attending Morehouse College and since she lived in Texas it was extra security knowing that she could hop on a plane at a moment's notice to get to him if she needed to.

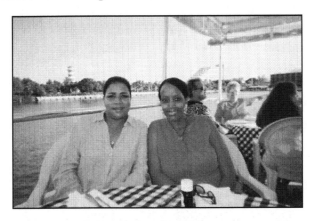

TJ and me in the Bahamas

TJ and I had so many travel experiences that we could write a book about it, but there were two trips that I will never forget. The first trip in my mind was the trip to Los Angeles after my stepsister Kim died. I didn't want to take that trip alone. TJ met my sister on an earlier visit so she was more than happy to come with me. Kim's mom Marolyn was happy that I was coming and maybe in a lot of ways it was like still having Kim. Marolyn and I formed a mother & daughter relationship and with my mother being deceased and now Kim, it was natural for us to gravitate towards one another. When I met all of Kim's family, everyone was so shocked to meet me because although they knew about me they did not realized how much we looked alike. Kim died from complications with her liver, caused by sickle cell disease. It was hard for me to digest. Like I said earlier, when it came to sickle cell whatever happened to me also happened to Kim and vice versa. The whole thought of her dying shook me to my very core. As I was on the plane headed to California, I thought about how permanent death was. You leave this stage of life forever and although I'm a believer and expect to go to heaven, I don't know if death is how I want to get there. Staying around until Jesus comes back sounds like a much better option. I can't say that I was sad that Kim died, because I knew how hard the battle was. On the other hand, she had such a love for life and the people around her. I know that she wanted to live and I wondered why not me. I was the one so tired of fighting. I was the war torn soldier not her. When I looked down into her casket and saw myself, there were so many thoughts running through my head. I remember very little about the service because I was reconciling things in my mind. Here I was with my sister's family while they mourn and all I could think about was myself. It was a sad day for me. I was so conflicted, on one hand I wanted to get back home and just give up and on the other hand I wanted to fight for my life.

The second flight that I will always remember occurred when I was on my way back home. TJ and I boarded the plane and sat back not saying anything to one another until something happened. I felt a large pop inside of my head. Oh God, I was so scared and immediately I thought that the brain aneurysm had ruptured. I knew it was there for nearly six or seven years, but the doctor said it was too small to take the risk of surgery. We were supposed to be watching it but we didn't. I turned to TJ in tears and she called over the flight attendant. I pulled out my pain medicine and assured them that I would be ok. I asked myself, is this how it will end? I was so scared because I watched my mom become someone who had to rely on others for everything. As strong as she was, if she couldn't get better I had no chance if that is what was happening to me. I always hoped that if it ever ruptured I would die immediately. The doctors told us that my mother bled in her brain for about three days before she came in for medical attention. They were amazed at her ability to withstand the pain that she endured prior to coming to the hospital. I remember how bad her head was hurting but it wasn't until she started vomiting that she went in. The memory of that was overtaking me and was causing me the most fear that I had faced to that point.

We finally made it back home and TJ went on to Texas. I called the doctor and he scheduled a MRI. I had a sinus infection and something related to that is what caused the pop. Because I suspected the aneurysm, they took a look at it and I was referred to a neurologist. The one that originally diagnosed it was in Texas, so we had to request my files from him. Once the new doctor had something to compare it with, it was plain to see that it had increased in size and was now much more of a threat. I was going to need surgery. Now I had a ticking time bomb in my head and my desire to die was really close to becoming a reality. After pondering my options and weighing the risk I made the decision to address this issue head on, but I knew I couldn't do it on my own. It was not fair to place all of the concern on Candis and I needed to move back to Texas. Candis' job was based in Atlanta and they don't have a base in Dallas so she would have to commute if she moved back with me. There were some tough decisions that needed to be made and how was this going to work out for us? All of my family was in Texas and I couldn't fight this like a one-man army. I needed a strong support system, so that if anything went wrong Candis and Jessica wouldn't be left to deal with it alone. TJ's son was now a student at Morehouse College and he wanted to get his own apartment. TJ and Candis had known each other for many years and he was family. We all talked about it and they decided to become roommates. She wouldn't be there often because she was coming back to Texas with me. She just needed a place to crash whenever she needed to be in Atlanta to start her work week. If she had to be at work early on Tuesday morning she would fly in on Monday and stay at the apartment in Atlanta so she would be there for work the next day. I gave them all of my furniture and we moved in with my sister and her family. She just had a baby right before I came so I was able to help her out until it was time for me to have my surgery. I am seven years older than she and before I moved in, we didn't really have a very close relationship. We both knew however that if we ever needed one another we could count on each other. Our mother had always instilled the importance of family in us. My sister now had four children and she and her husband had a large home and it accommodated us without it feeling cramped.

I had several consultations because the mouth of the aneurysm was almost too wide to perform a procedure that would keep them from having to cut into my head to repair it. I really needed to have the aneurysm coiled, because they could do that by accessing my brain through a large artery and releasing little coils into the aneurysm, which would block any further blood flow and eliminate the possibility of it rupturing. Earlier I spoke of the mouth of the aneurysm and what I meant by that is, it was too wide to hold the coiling in place. I had to undergo two procedures. The first one closed the mouth of it by creating a sort of fence with holes big enough for the device that releases the coils to go through. It's very technical but it was necessary in order for them to do the second procedure, which was placing the coils inside of the aneurysm. Both procedures inadvertently caused me to have a pain crisis. My entire family, including cousins and friends, was at the hospital praying for me and cheering me on. Some of them I never expected to be there. It was the most heartwarming time of my life. Knowing that I had that kind of support pulled me through. It was the toughest battle to date.

Getting What I Had Always Wanted

I think the fact that I was facing the same fate as my mother caused my father great concern. He was very upset by what happened to her and even though he was remarried and living in California he would visit her every time he came to Texas. He also attended her funeral and sat on the front row. I was in the hospital and they let me out for a few hours in order to attend the funeral. My dad grabbed my wheelchair and rolled me all the way to the front row and parked me in front of himself. That is how he ended up on the front row. He started keeping in touch and attempting to reconcile our relationship. When he found out how much I had endured he was truly sorry that he was so self- absorbed during the years that Kim and I needed him. I now had a healthy father/daughter relationship with him. While I was living with my sister he came and visited us for three weeks. He celebrated his 68th birthday with us and his grandchildren and great grand. It was a visit that was well overdue, but so necessary for me. I was on a plane to be by his side when he passed away. He had lots of regrets and God allowed him to reach out to his children and hopefully each of us took advantage of his attempt and received whatever may have been missing due to his absence. He was so proud of who I had become and being validated by my father felt great.

Time to Live Again

Several months after getting clearance that everything was done, I moved out of my sister's house and got my own place. Candis and Jessica moved out much earlier than I did. Candis now had an apartment in Dallas and in Atlanta and she was still commuting. I started to do some mystery shopping. Nobody could believe it. Finally something got me out of the house on a regular basis. I was known for loving to be at home and I can still stay home for days and weeks at a time and have no desire to leave the house. I think it's a contentment that I learned from having to be in the hospital so much. But more than loving being home, I loved role playing and undercover work. For me it felt like being a private investigator. I worked for over twenty mystery shopping companies and I was getting calls asking me to do special shops. It was pretty exciting, but it didn't pay much. I didn't care because I was having fun.

Even my husband and I were thinking about getting back together. In order to consider getting back with him I had to go on a fast. He always held a special place in my heart but I understood that too much had happened to us and unless God ordained our union it would be a fatal mistake for us to ever live together as husband and wife. Even though I felt like that, I never sought to divorce him even when it was obvious that he had moved on. I didn't want to get back together with him but God began to speak to me concerning our relationship and showing me that He would restore it. I reluctantly allowed him back into my life and it came at a time when Candis was getting tired of commuting. She saw that there was a good possibility that we would get back together so she used it as an opportunity to see if maybe we could all move back to Atlanta. Candis is very self sufficient and why she always wants me near is anybody's guess. It could be because of the bond that Jessica and I have or she wants to spend as much time with me as possible. We are constantly bumping heads, but it's our crazy life. After talking it over with my husband we felt it could possibly be a great way to start over fresh, so we decided that we would make the move.

Back to Atlanta

The lease was up on both of Candis' apartments and my brother took over the lease on mine so we packed up and we headed to Atlanta. We found a house that would accommodate us, so Candis would feel as though she still had her privacy and Jessica would have her own space. It wasn't anything spectacular, but since Phillip and I were both retired it was perfect because we had plans on traveling. It wasn't long before my sister and her family moved back to Atlanta as well. She lived here earlier as well and it was her husband's hometown. They found a home that was on the street right behind me, or shall I say I found it for them. It felt really good knowing that we had our own little village of support. Jessica would still be around her cousins and actually be more like their sister. They were all around the same age except for my sister's oldest daughter who is a teenager. The rest of them are little stair steps and Jessica fit right in the middle.

I tried really hard to remember that now that I was living with my husband, I couldn't continue to live like I was alone. That meant getting up and combing my hair and putting some clothes on. Getting out of my pajamas was a real sacrifice. It became apparent that this was going to take some work. I wasn't going to work at it if he wasn't and I guess I expected God to do all of the work. I can only compare it to Abraham and Sarah and how God promised them a child. If you know that story, then you know a whole lot of stuff happened before they got that promise.

Anyway, without putting all my business out there, although it's a little late for that, Phillip was gone before the year was out. We just didn't anticipate the work we would have to put into this marriage. The crazy thing is, I haven't given up hope as of today that is.

Something keeps haunting me. Why am I back in Atlanta? The first time I came here to die. The second time I came here for a fresh start. No matter why I came I feel as though God orchestrated it. There is a reason that I am here and it has everything to do with my destiny and my purpose.

Dealing with Regrets

Now I was dealing with another failure and it was so unnecessary. I was the one with the spiritual insight and I still blew it. Lord when will I learn how to go beyond my wants, my needs and my desires? That is why I can't stay satisfied. That is why when things get hard I want to give up and throw in the towel. You would think that Jessica would have taught me the joy of extending myself. Now all I can think about is poor me. My health isn't getting any better and now I'm turning 45. To most people that means nothing, but for me it's one more statistic to overcome. I have now reached the age of the average life expectancy of a female with sickle cell disease. When will these highs and lows cease. Why can't I just die and let it be over. I know that I keep going back and forth about if I want to live or not. Stop this insanity that is taking over my thoughts. Why am I so broken? Why can't I grab a zest for life again? Help me Lord. Please help me. This is way too much for me to bear. I can't fight this battle alone. The people around me are counting on me so they don't know I'm about to give up. Stop this torment Lord, bring me help or let me die.

I am the happiest when I am helping others, but now I need help. I can't show it, I can't say it, so how is anyone supposed to know it. That is my dilemma, how do I break the silence? How do I share my struggle? Is there anyone who will understand? More so, is there anyone who will care?

Maybe I'm not the only one who felt like that. I created an online support page called the Advocacy Group for Adults with Sickle Cell Anemia and within two weeks or so I had over five hundred fans of the page. I was shocked that there were people out there that might be like me.

Nicole Williams was one of the first people to draw on me from my very soul. She was a young lady around the same age as my daughter and she had sickle cell along with her twin sister. Prior to me starting the page, Nicole's sister died. It was six months later that her mother died. I could feel the devastation in her. Maybe it was because I was so broken and sensitive at the time. She always maintained a tough exterior, so there was nothing that she said that pulled at me it was a sense of connection. It could have been the helplessness that we both shared or maybe the battle that had us holding on for dear life all the while wanting to lose our grip. Whatever it was, it bonded us for life. I can't remember exactly what was said, but she indicated she wouldn't mind me being her mom and I told her she could have me with one warning. I was a "Smother Mother". She didn't mind that at all, she could probably use a little bit of smothering. After several online chats she went into the hospital with a pain crisis and I would text her to stay in touch with what was going on with her. If she was hurting too much to respond, I instructed her to reply with "k." That would be my indication that she was really having a tough time. Over time we really did become mother and daughter. Candis had a tendency to get a little jealous when other people tried to get that close to me, but with Nicole it was different. She may have been able to see that I needed Nicole as much as she needed me.

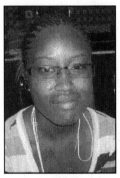

Nicole Williams

The Song

Now that I was beginning to meet others with sickle cell, I knew that this thing was bigger than me. During my darkest hours, I always referred to sickle cell as being a battle and if that was true we all had to be soldiers. I don't know if I went to bed thinking about that or not, but one morning I woke up and sat straight up in my bed because I heard these words ringing in my ears. I grabbed my pad and pen and began to write what I thought was a poem. I wrote:

I've been fighting this thing, for much too long
And I just can't fight this, on my own.
I've been trying to speak and my voice is too low
But If I can't tell them, then how will they know.
My back's against the wall, and I'm going down way too fast
If something doesn't happen, then I'm not going to last
They don't understand, I'm 'bout to let it all go
I'm tired of being strong, and they don't even really know.
This thing is pulling on me, and I'm down on the ground
I'm gonna need some help, to turn this thing around.
I'm not facing this giant, all by myself
'Cause God sent me soldiers, just to give me some help
They're fighting for me, 'cause at times I get weak
When the pain is taking over, I just can't speak.
I need some soldiers, in this battle with me
I need some soldiers, who will help them to see
I need some soldiers, in this battle with me
I need some front line, front line soldiers with me

The more I read it the more it sounded like it could be a song. I tried to get Candis to take a look at it but she was too busy. I tried to put a melody to it but it sounded like an old Negro spiritual, so I was at my wits end. This was exactly the message that I need to express to those who were around me, but would they ever get a chance to see these words?

Then I thought about my niece Cheryl in Los Angeles. She is a rapper and she goes by the name Mecca Dawn, but she also has a beautiful singing voice. I called her up and told her what was going on and we had a very interesting conversation. She had been going through some spiritual house cleaning shall I say and she felt like she needed to do some charity work. Sounded like God was up to something and He was. I emailed her the lyrics that evening and when I woke up the next morning there was an attachment from her in my email inbox. She found the beats and sang the song in a way that excited me so much, that I called everybody I knew. That song was my own personal anthem. Not only was it my anthem, it ignited me to take my online support off line. People needed some real advocacy and awareness of their battle. Maybe this song could persuade them to reach out for help. Maybe if people knew this battle was too tough to endure, they would help.

The SCD Soldier Network, Inc.

It was time to make it happen. For the very first time in my life I finally had real hope that my suffering was going to impact the world more than my healing ever did. I felt God calling me to build this network of support, where it would be safe for people to say they needed help. Where there was a sea of supporters waiting to meet their needs, where there were people dedicated to helping those with Sickle Cell Disease. SCD Soldier Network would be that place. We would hold three-day boot camps and train advocates. We would create a speakers bureau so that those who wanted to speak about sickle cell could be trained, so that the community was speaking with a united voice. Even people who never knew anything about sickle cell could learn and offer their support and help us to bring more awareness to the blood disorder. I wanted us to shine the spotlight on those who are battling the disease and making great strides in perseverance and are successful in things that would bring hope to the younger generations to come. The vision was so clear that I couldn't do anything but say yes. God I will resonate throughout my being. Purpose and destiny was reigning supreme and I didn't care what I had to do to make this dream a reality, I would be doing it until they laid my body down.

I knew it would take money and I didn't have any so since I did taxes during tax season, whatever money I could make from that I would put toward the vision. Most of the work would take years to yield results, so what could I do right away? We could build a website that would stand as a recruiting station so we could build a database. Then we could support awareness campaigns by providing volunteers to help organizations who were already established. We could also highlight the efforts of our front-line soldiers (that term is reserved for those who are actively battling sickle cell and/or helping to bring awareness to the disease). Before we could really make an impact we needed to change the way people with sickle cell are perceived. We are not helpless and we are not weak. The average person would be hard pressed to deal with the battle of sickle cell. We are now living longer so in addition to our poster child, we are going to need a new image, an image of strength and endurance. I suggest it's a soldier.

People Who Are Making the Vision Happen

There is no way I could make this happen by my self. I may be the visionary, but I'm going to need some help. There would be no Soldier Network without the help of Mr. Dan Moore of APEX Museum of Atlanta, GA. I was referred to him because he was working on a documentary about bone marrow transplants and the need for more African American donors. He wanted to include sickle cell as one of the diseases that would benefit from increased donors and I was told he was looking for people with a story to tell. Perfect timing for me because, I was finally ready to scream my story from the rooftop. I met with Mr. Moore and by the end of our discussion he vowed to help me make SCD Soldier Network a reality. He showed me things that would have cost me thousands of dollars, without his advice because I was not equipped to do some of the necessary paperwork. This man has encouraged and supported me and to this day I still don't know why. He is also the reason that I am telling my story in this book. He saw something in me that I don't know that I've seen yet. I have only seen him face to face a few times, but each time I do he inspires me to reach further and do more - To finish out the rest of my life where the world can see. I pray that one day I can be that for somebody else, because it's from my heart when I say he has challenged me in a way that I will never lose hope again. I will run my race and finish my course because of Mr. Moore.

The Work of A SCD Soldier

Finding sponsorship and building the database is going to be the key to our success and with this being a national group my flight benefits are coming in handy. Until we begin to generate funding that will allow us to train more advocates and put outreach programs into place, I am taking it to the streets and I am reaching out everywhere that I can for help. There are some people that I must mention because without them I don't know which way I would have gone and how far off of course I would be. Some of these people have become my confidants, my advisors and my prayer partners. There is no way that I can mention all of the people who have crossed my path and left a lifelong impression on me. This list consists of those who are supporting me right now in such a way that I would be remiss if I did not mention them.

Helen Mitchell - Sickle Cell Mom & Advocate

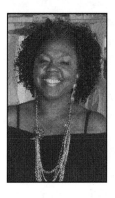

I met Helen on twitter in the latter part of 2009. Her daughter Kameron Moore-Mitchell who is a rapper by the stage name TheSekondElement was having a fundraising event. This event was for the benefit of children in Northern California with sickle cell disease. She was hoping to raise enough money to pay for several of them to go to sickle cell camp. I was very impressed by how young Kameron was and although she has sickle cell, she was also an advocate making things happen. After following her tweets I realized that her mother was also on twitter and the dialog between the two of them was much like my daughter and I. I started following Helen and there was an instant bond. Two mothers who had reared very strong young ladies who knew how to work our nerves. I say that jokingly because both of our daughters are outspoken and what comes up comes out. They are free spirits and have little room for nonsense. Just like Candis and I, it didn't matter that we were polar opposites the love was evident. I started tweeting with Helen and soon found out she was on FaceBook as well. I became her FaceBook friend and the rest is history. I don't know if social media ever set out to connect strangers in hopes that they would find a common ground to build a friendship, but if so Helen and I could be their poster child. I was supposed to meet Helen at her daughter's event but I ended up having a sickle cell crisis and was admitted into the hospital. It wasn't until six months later that I had the chance to meet her face to face in Los Angeles at the Be Sickle Smart Empowerment Event. It was the final step to solidifying our friendship and I think that Helen is as much of a friend as I have ever had. I talk to Helen nearly every day and she is someone who I can vent to, cry on and celebrate with. She lives many miles from me, but I always feel just a phone call away. Thanks Kameron for the incredible work that you are doing and for leading me to your mother.

Nita Thompson – Sickle Cell Mom & Advocate

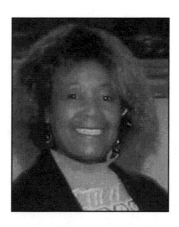

I went to Los Angeles in order to record the SCD Soldier Anthem and when I told Helen that I was going, she told me to be sure to contact a lady by the name of Nita Thompson. When I arrived, Nicole picked me up from the airport and took me to my hotel. She actually stayed with me the entire time and provided all of my transportation. I got settled in and made the hundred phone calls that I needed to make in order to connect with some of the potential soldiers that I had in CA. One of those calls went out to Nita Thompson. She not only was an advocate for sickle cell, she was on a full-scale campaign for more African Americans to donate blood, stem cells and bone marrow. This lady blew my mind. She met me at the hotel and I invited her up so that we could talk in detail. As she began to talk, I told her that I had to get our conversation on video. I pulled out my old video camera from the 1990's and started recording. She was passionate about what she was doing and she was one of the most aggressive people that I have ever met. Nita has been such a major help to me because she began to change my language. She is teaching me how loose the word "trying" from my vocabulary and anybody who knows her, knows that when she comes, she's coming to do business. I know that she can be a little too aggressive for some people, but when it comes to sickle cell awareness she could teach a whole lot of us how to make things happen. I love Nita and above all, I know that even when she is giving me corrective criticism it is coming from a place of love and support. She has spoken nothing but success over my life and the life of SCD Soldier Network. Thank you Nita, for being true to who you are, and I'll see you on the frontlines.

Velvet Brown Watts – Sickle Cell Mom & Advocate

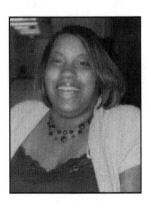

When the local sickle cell association in Tulsa lost its state funding they closed their doors. Velvet and other citizens affected by sickle cell in the area wanted to do something, because they were left without any representation. Velvet has a son with sickle cell and she knew that the families needed help. She helped to spearhead the organization that now serves the families in that area. Velvet and I were both attempting to assist Dominique Friend, a sickle cell advocate and author to form a coalition. When she found out that I was on board she contacted me to find out more about what the SCD Soldier Network was about. She began to question me about the name because she had concerns about the implications of sounding like a militant group. Her line of questions challenged me and it caused me to develop some real objectives. I don't think that I expected to be friends with her, but I sure am glad that we did become friends. Velvet is very clear about what needs to happen in the sickle cell community and her expertise in developing an organization on top of her background in social work, makes her a definite asset. Beyond being supporting advocates we are developing a friendship. The last time that I was in the hospital, I had a situation that happened with one of my nurses and I was very upset about it, plus I was on a lot of narcotics which elevated the imbalance of my emotions. It was a serious situation where my nurse purposely withheld my pain medication because she was not comfortable with the amount that I was receiving. I was lucent enough to advocate for myself and bring closure to the issue but I was upset that this very thing was being experienced everyday by those hospitalized with sickle cell disease. Velvet happened to call me at the end of my ordeal and I was very emotional and looking back, I know I must have sounded like an intoxicated lunatic to her. Velvet was so enduring and wanted to hear through the craziness exactly how I was handling the situation. My whole focus was on all of the people who didn't know how to advocate for themselves under conditions where they are in pain and are on a large amount of narcotics. I was a babbling nut that day and Velvet stayed on the phone with me until all of my ranting and raving ceased. I will never be able to thank her for enduring that, because if someone else would have been on the other end of that conversation I don't think they would have known exactly what to do. My friend, prayer partner, front line soldier and future partner in advocacy I am truly grateful that you entered my life.

LaToya Ford-Tucker – Sickle Cell Mom & Advocate

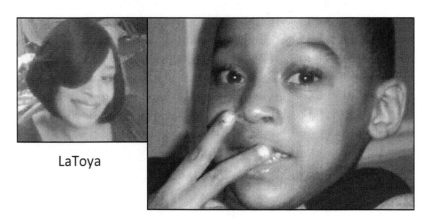

LaToya

LaToya's son Zyyir

Velvet introduced me to a young lady by the name of LaToya Ford-Tucker. She lived in Atlanta and was looking for support for her family. Her eight year-old son Zyyir had been having a rough time lately and had been out of school for months due to complications from sickle cell disease. The hospital bills were piling up and there was no help that she could find. After I spoke with LaToya it was like an eye-opening experience. I was shocked to find out that the kids who battle sickle cell weren't that far ahead of the adults. I guess I thought that things were really progressing for kids with the disorder and it was their adult counterparts who had fallen through the cracks in the system. There is just so much work to do and I know that it will probably be plenty of work left for the future generations. That is why I decided that we needed to include programs and services for kids into our mission. Finding out the problem that teens are having transitioning into to the adult system was even more reason to extend the organization beyond supporting only adults with sickle cell disease. LaToya told me that her son was beginning to feel as though he was different and he didn't like knowing that he was. My heart was breaking because when I was a kid I don't remember feeling like that. Whenever my mind was quiet I thought about Zyyir and my sleep was not peaceful until I decided that we would make being different something to be proud of for Zyyir. I talked to LaToya and then I talked to him and we made it official. Zyyir Tucker would head up our Tiny Soldiers division. He was elated and so was I. We were doing more than appeasing a young boy. We are training a future advocate and our next leader. LaToya has rolled up her sleeves and helps out whenever she is needed. She is in the military so we are hoping to gain the support of the armed forces through a "Soldiers Helping Soldiers" campaign. Together we will build up the soldier count in GA and make our home base our strongest area.

Veronica Very

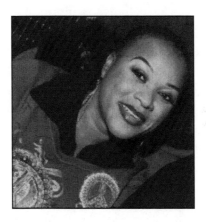

Veronica Very was the first person to ever go to SCD Soldier Network's website and call me. She lives in Seattle, WA and when she called me, I could feel the desperation in her voice. She had been to the website looking for help for her daughter Ashle'. It wasn't what she said so much that pulled at me, it was knowing, she felt alone in a town that in her opinion offered little help for those with sickle cell. It is when a person reaches that level of hopelessness that you know there is a potential for God to do something. I didn't know exactly what would happen with her or her daughter, but I knew that she had a "Lord, send me" in her belly. If I had to describe what I felt, I would have to say I was feeling as though she was drawing from me. Her spirit was connecting with mine much like Mary and Elizabeth of the Bible. Even now whenever we have our 'what we call' two-part conversations something spiritual happens. Her presence makes my vision jump up and down in the womb of my spirit. It was not long after our initial conversation that I noticed that she was on FaceBook and she had started a "Break Sickle Silence" support page and was in the process of starting her own foundation. I was joyous when I saw it, because I knew God was in the midst of what was going on. Veronica is a woman of faith and she is full of substance and operates at a level of excellence. She has a unique ability to get people talking about the disease and how it has affected their lives. She may be new to the world of National Advocacy, but God is promoting her quickly. Veronica and her new organization will be my first official partner when we celebrate the launching of Very Bright Foundation in September 2010.

Lakiea Bailey – Front Line Soldier & Advocate

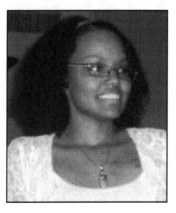

Lakiea was another person who was attempting to assist with the coalition and that is how I met her. She has sickle cell and is in medical school here in Georgia. I was so impressed by her knowledge of the disease and everything related to it. When I finally met her face-to-face I knew that her small stature and soft voice was not an indicator of the giant that she really was. Due to the fact that she is in medical school and also battling sickle cell, she was not always available, but she always offered her knowledge. I count on her as an advisor when it comes to forming this organization. She is the one person who connects a lot of the dots that have been drawn for SCD Soldier Network. She is responsible for introducing me to Mr. Dan Moore and Mrs. Tina Kay Hughes. She is one of my core members and though we don't get to talk very much, there was no way I was leaving her out of my story. She has been there since the beginning and I am hoping that when she graduates she can be a little more active, but right now she is an excellent example of what you can achieve in spite of your battle with sickle cell disease. I have a mountain of respect for Lakiea and she makes me proud.

Tina Kay Hughes – Front Line Soldier, Author & Advocate

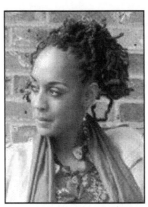

Lakiea was working to help Tina facilitate a book signing in Atlanta and that is how we met. I was asked to help bring people to her book reading and signing. She wrote a book and was on a promotional tour. I had not really tapped into the Atlanta market yet so LaToya and I came to one of her book readings at the Sickle Cell Foundation of GA patient support group meeting. We came as representatives of SCD Soldier Network. Tina was a very sweet young lady and her mother was right by her side. I knew that if my mother were still alive and well she would be by my side just like that. I was in love with the image that I saw and after the reading I was happy to actually speak with both of them. She had signed up as a front line soldier so I decided to highlight her on the website and include her book on one of the hand out's that I include in a package that I provide whenever I do recruiting drives. Several weeks later she called me because she wanted to know if perhaps we could coordinate our tours. I was attempting to schedule two recruiting drives a month and we both felt it was a good way partner up. At my recruiting drive there are usually three elements that I like to include. 1) I like to have a front line soldier who is doing something to bring awareness to the disease. 2) I usually have a person who can speak about the need for blood, stem cell and bone marrow donations. 3) I like to have a representative of a sickle cell organization in that city to speak about the services and programs that they offer. Since Tina wanted to join the tour, it would give me my front line soldier and plus I wouldn't be hosting these events alone. It was perfect timing and like anything else, timing is everything. I haven't known Tina very long but we enjoy talking and supporting each other and by working together I hope to build a closer friendship with her. I am expecting our relationship to be one that will be filled with fun, laughter, support and success.

Front Line Organizations

There are several organizations and/or groups that I want to recognize because their founders and organizers are front line soldiers who battle sickle cell disease, treat those with it and/or advocate for others affected by it. You can find many of their support pages on facebook. They have caught a hold of the vision and have joined SCD Soldier Network in order to strengthen our cords. These are our commanders in advocacy and I salute them.

Akiim DeShay – BlackBoneMarrow.com

Alice Obedi – CESCA- Kenya

Andrell Wilson – SCD Soldier Network

Annette Delgado – Mindful Heart for Sickle Cell

Ashle' Johnson – Very Bright Foundation

Ayoola Olajide – SCD Journal – Ikorodu, Lagos

Byron Johnson – Colorado Sickle Cell Association

Chaznee Brown - Sickle Cell Anemia Foundation (SCAF) of East Bay

Cheryl Zachery – SCD Soldier Anthem (Artist: Mecca Dawn)

Christine Tyson – Increase Entertainment

Cynthia Uduebor – Otis Uduebor Foundation

Dan Moore, Sr. – Marrow For Life –Author, In Search of a Match

DeLita Rose-Daniels – Citizens for Quality Sickle Cell Care, Inc.

Dominique Friend – Author of Sickle

Emmanuel Oyelere – Rural Sickle Cell Group

Eric Kirkwood – SCDAA Uriel Owens Chapter

Esther Agbaje – SCANCA Patient Support Group

Fiona Howe – Sickle Cell Self Care

Gori Dean - MyLifeMoon

Hope Wright – TWSDLife (Twisted – Teens With Sickle Cell Disease)

Ishia Washington-Gattis – Author of Meet Camdem (A Children's Book about SCD)

Jose Guevara, Chiropractor – Premier Health & Rehab, LLC

Kameron Moore-Mitchell – TheSekondElement at KAMMsTheAce.com

Kisha Braswell – Medical Educator / Program Coordinator for the sickle SAFE program

LaMonte Forthun – TEAM (Teach, Educate and Medicate) Sickle Cell

Myiesha Demery – Sickle Cell Sistahood

Nita Thompson – AA Blood Drive and Marrow Registry 4 SC Awareness

Phyllis Bazen – Creator of a SCD Stress Study

Tanya Gentry – Sickle Cell Disease Association of San Diego

Tina Kay Hughes – Author of Walking In Your Season

Teonna Woolford – Breaking The Silence And The Sickle Cycle

Thelma Nartekie Nartey – Ecobank Ghana Limited

Tiffany Zachery – CrisRoy Zach Entertainment

Tosin Ola – Sickle Cell Warrior

Traci Adams – Hope Cells

Velvet Brown-Watts – Supporters of Families with Sickle Cell

Veronica Very – Break Sickle Silence & Very Bright Foundation

Special Thanks

There are some who have come and are gone, but they are still an essential part of my story. My story has not been told in its entirety and one day I hope to do that, but for now I'm thankful for the opportunity to have shared a piece of what has led me to the formation of SCD Soldier Network, Inc.

I want to thank all of the people who have joined us and are a part of our database for having patience while the process continues. I thank the soldiers who have volunteered and participated in awareness events. I thank all of my recruiters who keep spreading the word. I thank my family for getting involved and finding out what I have been up to. To the organizations that have opened their minds to the idea that the SCD Soldier Network could actually strengthen their organization. To the National Office of Sickle Cell Disease Association Of America, thank you for helping me to reach out to the local chapters and for affording me the opportunity to gain more experience in the area of advocacy.

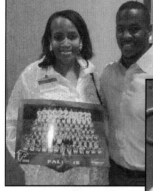

Eric Coleman
Atlanta Falcons

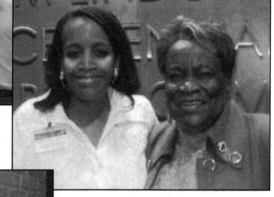

Jean Brannan,
Sickle Cell Foundation of Atlanta

Phyllis, and Dan Moore,

Dedication

My story is dedicated to my mother and father, whom God saw fit to use as vessels to bring me into the universe. It is also dedicated to the fallen soldiers, who have lost their battle with sickle cell disease. May they all rest in peace knowing that their existence served a higher purpose.

www.SCDSoldiernetwork.com

Sickle Cell Warriors

Becoming Self-Empowered

Meet Tosin Ola

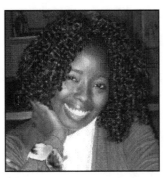

Hello my wonderful warriors. It's time for a heart 2 heart.

"When I was a child, I knew nothing about sickle cell. The only thing I knew about it was what my mom had told me from what the doctors told her. It wasn't until my teen years that I started reading about sickle cell on my own. Even then, whenever I fell sick, I turned into a younger version of myself, needing my mom at the bedside 24/7."

"It wasn't until I went off to college that I had to take a level of responsibility for my disease. Even then, I still was not eating right, or following the basic principles of sickle cell. I still relied heavily on what my doctors told me to do and did no research of my own. I lived from one crises to another, with daily pain and relied heavily on narcotics."

"My turning point occurred in 2001. I was living on my own 800 miles from home, and had gone into sickle cell crises. I went to the hospital, and my crises was so bad that I ended up being admitted. I knew that Morphine reduced my respirations, and yet, when the nurse came with a PCA of

Morphine, I said nothing. I was in a lot of pain, and just wanted it to be over. The nurse set the Morphine PCA to have a 'maintenance dose', which means that every hour, regardless of what my state was, I would get 5 mg of Morphine. I felt myself getting tired and sleepy, and still, I said nothing.

In the middle of the night, I became unresponsive, not breathing, and had to be rushed to the ICU. Fortunately, they were able to give me Narcan to reverse the effects of the Morphine, but my health took a downturn during that admission and I almost died. That was my turning point."

"See in that situation, I could blame the hospital, doctors and nurses. But the expert in the room was me. I had sickle cell for 21 years at that point, and I knew my body. I knew that Morphine would reduce my breathing, but I said nothing to the nurse or anyone. I didn't empower myself with my voice, *and I almost died*."

"Last year, a sickle cell warrior died because of iron overload. She knew that her iron was high, and that at a Hemoglobin count of 7 she could manage with the transfusion, but she accepted the blood transfusion anyway."

"Last month, my friend was in the hospital in crises, having pains in his leg and knee. The doctors wanted to do a biopsy of his knee. He knew that the pain was related to his sickle cell, and not anything was wrong with his knee but he said nothing. They did the biopsy, and his knee became infected at the aspiration point. He was hospitalized for an additional week because of that infection."

"Are you beginning to see a pattern here?"

"Please be a self empowered advocate. I know that you are in pain, when you go to the hospital, but that is not an excuse to keep silent. Silence kills! No one knows your body more than you, and you do not have to accept every single drug and treatment that they try to foist on you in the hospital. I'm not saying be cantankerous and noncompliant, but I am telling you to ask questions, make sure you understand the full picture, do your research, and do not just do something because that is what the doctors are telling you to do."

"My doctor never told me about the diet modifications that I can make to prevent crises. My doctor never told me about Nicosan, an herbal remedy that has kept me crises and pain free for over 2 years. My doctor never told me about the energy boost that I can get from Arginine. My doctor never told me that Melatonin can help with insomnia or that Fish oil can help with depression."

"Do you see the pattern here? All the improvements to my health and condition have been because I researched it, empowered myself and found out what works for my body. The docs are following a template in treating you, and they are not personally invested in your outcome. **THIS IS YOUR LIFE!** It is not your mom's, your spouse's or your doctors. This is your life, and you have to take ownership of it."

"God has gifted you with a brilliant mind. Technology has given us Google. There is no excuse for not researching every single little thing you need to know about sickle cell. Stop being a victim of the medical system. Stop relying on your parents or family to help you manage your condition. There is no excuse for ignorance—not in this day and age. **So please, I beg you, for the sake of your own life, take ownership and become self-empowered. Become your own advocate, speak up, and take care of yourself!**"

http://sicklecellwarriors.com/sc-connected/

Meet Dr. Jide Sokoya

Nigerian
Obstetrician/Gynecologist

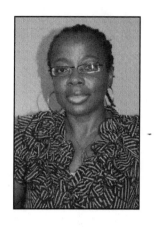

"I was 4 yrs old. The doctors initially thought I had appendicitis. My parents raised me just like my siblings without sickle cell disease. Growing up in Nigeria, I used to be out of school for ~ 6 months out of the year. Yes, I had SSD but no excuses allowed. School was important and I was expected to catch up with my classmates. When I wasn't sick I had to do everything everyone else did: cleaned the house, washed clothes, cooked, fetched water. Sounds easy right, but it actually wasn't. Cleaning the house involved scrubbing the walls and floors, washing clothes was done by hand, no washer and dryer. Cooking involved grinding red hot peppers by hand, using grinding stones, my hands would sting for hours, because I was pretty bad at it. Fetching water, sometimes involved waking up at 'ole dark thirty', as in the crack before the crack of dawn, walking for ~ an hour or more each way, sometimes waiting for ~ two or three hours in long lines. Walking back home with a bucket full of water on my head, all before breakfast. All these things were my parents teaching me discipline."

"I have always liked science, and was the geeky kid who would rather read the encyclopedia, than socialize. Don't get me wrong, I'm not antisocial! The human body intrigued me, plus I was always fascinated by people who were different; It was always easy for me to make friends with the 'outsiders' 'cause' I felt like one."

"My typical work day starts at 8 am. I work 24 hour shifts covering several different areas - Clinic, seeing patients in the office, - Labor and delivery- laboring patients, including performing cesarean sections. I also cover Triage (the emergency room), which may include anything from treating pregnant women with colds, to performing emergency surgery on a patient with an ectopic pregnancy (pregnancy in the tube). Consults from inpatients and patient transfers from other hospitals also keep me pretty busy. My job involves being a compassionate, caring physician, being diplomatic, multitasking and fielding problems. It is highly stressful and requires a great deal of concentration. Honestly, I am not always the aforementioned descriptive, especially when achy, or exhausted. Patience, is not my strongest suit, I'm working on it!"

"I try to stay hydrated when working, eat healthy and take a ten or twenty minute power nap when I can. Sometimes I'm running for 24hrs straight because so much is going on."

"Medical school classes started at 7.30am till about 6pm Monday through Friday. I was in the ER several times and had a few hospitalizations. I figured out I wasn't cut out to be a Pediatrician because I would always catch whatever they had. My friends were pretty cool with my SSD, and would help me catch up with school work. The Residents and Attending physicians were also pretty nice and would make sure I was well taken care of."

"Residency was different I was now a real physician working 24-40 hr days. Not all colleagues were sympathetic to working extra hours to cover a sick doc. My friends came through by starting IVs in the call room or in my apartment when it wasn't too busy, or I was off. The nurses and anesthesiologists would give me pain meds sometimes, because I did not have a regular physician. Probably all illegal but hey they got me through."

"I'll say it's very challenging! Between work, port flushes and doctors appointments I feel like I have 2 full time jobs! When I come home from work in the morning, everything hurts. I usually would take Oxycodone + a muscle relaxant+ a heating pad for my legs and rest during the day if I can. I have a Gastroenterologist and a Hematologist/Oncologist that I see every few months- I keep my appointments, drink plenty of water, try to eat as much unprocessed food as I can, take my medicine, well most of the time, and try to get as much rest as I can. The last one is actually very hard, I'm an insomniac and sleep whenever I can, which is during the day when I'm not working. I work two or three 24 hour shifts a week."

"I'm tired a lot of times because of my work schedule and taking narcotics, so I don't have a lot of time to socialize. I would like to be in a relationship with someone nice, who understands me and is considerate of me."

"Nine years ago I was diagnosed with cancer. Prayer, my friends, and family helped me through. My favorite sayings *'God never gives you more than you can handle'* and *'When you are going through hell, keep on going'* also give me the extra strength to keep on pushing."

"I am in pain EVERYDAY!!! My pain usually runs from a 3 to a 5 on a 10 pain scale. I do not and will not take narcotics when working, it's like driving drunk, so I just deal with it, or take Tramadol close to when I'm about to finish my shift, if it is really bad. Rarely if it is really, super bad; I'll take Toradol and have an IV started. Oxycodone, Toradol, Tramadol Folic acid/2 GI meds for ulcers/ Hydroxyurea/Cymbalta/Multivitamins."

"In 2001, I developed Non-Hodgkins Lymphoma, 6 months after starting Hydroxyurea (Now, I'm in complete remission). I do not know if the Hydroxyurea precipitated it, however my last hospital admission was in 2007. So I take it, because it works for me."

"If I could look back to the time I was fourteen I would tell my 14 year old self: 'life gets better.' "

Meet Tina Kay Hughes

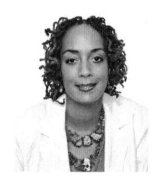

"I look at the world with a different set of eyes that see God's goodness in everything all around me. Despite the doctors' reports, x-rays, Cat scans and some days a body that is in constant turmoil; I still know in my heart that I am in this space at this particular time to make a difference in the lives of others. My plan is not always the right plan and makes me realize God planned long ago these, my days, for me. So I accept God's grace, mercy, love, and challenges as His way of using me to the benefit of and for all of His people."

"Are you living, or are you just existing?" I love this quote because over the past three years as Sickle Cell Disease has begun its attack against my body and mind, many days I feel like I am just here, existing. I think I am a type A personality, always needing order, a definitive plan, and structure. However, living with Sickle Cell there is no structure; your days are determined by your body."

"During my childhood, I lived like any other child—not knowing or feeling any difference between myself and other children. I played outside, participated in many sports and school activities and was an over achiever and often times found myself in positions of leadership. There were only two instances that I remember quite vividly as a child having pneumonia and receiving blood transfusions around the age of 8. The other time was in college, in a small town, where doctors did not know how to treat this disease. I had an awful urinary tract infection that caused me to urinate blood. The doctors sent me home to urinate overnight in a bag. By the time my mother rushed me home from college (a 2 hour drive) I needed a blood transfusion. My college days were extremely stressful and I spent many days in the University's infirmary every quarter during finals to receive IV fluids, to avoid hospitalization."

"I spent 10 years working in the insurance industry. I traveled all over the country. I was never sick during those years except for maybe 2 times. My last days as a claims adjuster, I could not carry out the basic functions of my position, so I was retired by my company as disabled."

"Never in a million years would I have imagined not being able to do simple things in my life. For instance, combing my hair, cooking a meal, driving myself, washing my hair and body, feeding myself, having children, and putting on my clothing just to name a few. Life is so precious and taken for granted until something in life causes you to pause and take account of what is really important and what things or issues are really worth being mad about, fighting for, and spending way too much energy on. Every day that I wake, I have to do things based on how my body feels for the day—it could mean I stay in bed all day, stay in the house all day, or actually go and have fun. I have no control and this drives me completely insane."

"It irritates me when people make off hand comments like, 'You don't look sick' or 'You look good are you sure you are sick.' The one thing I can control is my outward appearance and this is just a part of my personality, a need to be in control of something, and my appearance is the one thing I can control."

"Currently, I have bone infarcts all over my ribs, vascular necrosis in both shoulders (where the bones are slowly deteriorating), bursitis in my hips, blood clots in my stomach, complete loss of hearing in my right ear, and to be determined if I have lupus or rheumatoid arthritis in my hands and feet. I also contracted Hepatitis C due to blood transfusions in the 80's and early 90's. It takes about two hours every day that I wake for my body to respond to pain medication so I am able to move out of the bed. Despite, the goings on in my body, I feel many days like there is a terrorist in my body, waging war and I have no defense to stop it. I love my husband so much because he is always by my side as a best friend and whatever else he needs to be. My family and friends are always at my beck and call to do whatever is needed. Without the love of family and friends I don't know that I could make it through some of my worst days."

"I've spent many days in the hospital. I am thankful that President Obama is calling, pushing, and putting into action a new health care plan. I worry about the ceiling on my health insurance policy, exorbitant amounts I pay for the deductible and out of pocket costs. I also worry about being dropped by my health insurance carrier because I have a chronic illness. These are the things that remain at the forefront of your mind when you are often ill. Whereas, if one has never suffered through any type of health issue or witnessed a loved one suffer, one cannot fully grasp the need for health care reform."

"I journal to help my mental state; I also, create and design jewelry as a release that is therapeutic for me. My writings have been compiled into a book to help others who have any type of struggles in life. The endorphins that are released during my therapeutic hobbies help the pain to subside for just a little while." See www.tinakay.net

"I have so much hope and faith that a cure will come to fruition soon for adults with Sickle Cell because a cure for children with Sickle Cell has already been discovered. They say the life expectancy for adults with Sickle Cell is approximately 40-50 years old. People living with Sickle Cell are like the forgotten few left alone to suffer in silence. There is very little attention given by the medical community to this disease. There is very few research dollars spent on SC Disease even though it is a global problem. It is also present in Portuguese, Spanish, French Corsicans, Sardinians, Sicilians, mainland Italians, Greeks, Turks and Cypriots. Sickle cell disease also appears in Middle Eastern countries and Asia. This is not a disease where I did something to contract it - I was born with this disease. My greatest fear is that I will not be able to do or see all the things in life I hope for before my life comes to an end."

"Not only does the African American community but the wider community remain quiet, clueless, and uneducated about SC Disease. I feel as if I have to be my own advocate, because no one else is speaking on my behalf nor is anyone going before the masses to draw attention to this disease like attention is given to other diseases. My hope is the larger community will put this disease on their radar, so healing and wholeness can begin to dwell in the lives of those with Sickle Cell."

For additional information concerning Sickle Cell visit the following websites:
http://www.sicklecellministries.org
http://sicklecell-ourvoice.blogspot.com/

Meet **Mrs. Bridgett DeShae' Wright-Willkie**

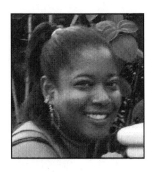

"I asked my mother, when I had my first crisis. She told me that when I was 3 years old, we were at my brother Phil's high school football game. I wet my clothes and that is what happened to be the trigger for what we now know, was my very 1st crisis. Since then, we would realize that every time I got wet, by swimming, getting caught in the rain or something as simple as sitting in the bath tub for too long. I would have these God awful pains and fits of crying out but there was no curve to grade the pain on. No one else in my entire family has SCD...I am the last of six children. My mom has four from her 1st marriage and two from my father. I went through this unpredictable pain whenever I got too cold, played too long or even from falling asleep on my arm the wrong way (you know when your arm falls asleep). Now this whole time, my mom thought that she was doing the right thing by taking me to my pediatrician, but all Dr. Parker would do is send me home with Children's Tylenol b/c he said that I had 'Growing Pains'! So that was my life from the age of

3 until they discovered that I had over 140 gallstones at the age of 17."

"So, here is where my second life began. Along with being told that I had to cut back on my daily intake of fried okra from Church's Chicken. I was hit with the diagnosis of having Sickle Cell Disease and that, at the time the average life expectancy was only 23 years old. I swore that I'd been given a 5 year death sentence. I went through all of the phases that one would go through after a life threatening diagnosis. At first, I was relieved to know that I wasn't crazy and that we finally had a name for my affliction. Then, I got mad after learning of the statistics on SCD. I started questioning my faith and wondered IF there was a God, what in the world it was that My parents did for me to wind up with it. I then went through a phase of researching and accepting it. I wanted to find out as much as possible. I wanted to meet as many other's with the disease. All that I had learned in life, no longer applied to me anymore. There was so much I wanted to accomplish growing up. Watching my mother work and raise six children basically on her own, I now know that it wouldn't be that simple for me to do the same. I was so desperate to remove myself from my little home town of Sanford, Florida. I did the unimaginable...I enlisted in the United States Air Force, I tried to sneak in but my high score on the ASVAB was my downfall, the job that I chose was Air Traffic Control. They had to test my blood under more stressful conditions and it sickled before they got it to the lab. They sent me back home but I still had to get away."

"I had a desire to go on to college and so I went to the local community college for a couple of semesters then I went to Tallahassee to pursue a degree in Architecture, from Florida Agricultural & Mechanical University. Once there, most likely from all of the stress of being on my own, I started getting sick more often. With Architecture, if you miss 1 day it takes you 2 days to make it up, now imagine how long it would take to make up for being in the hospital for 2 weeks. Okay, so I had to change my major and went for Journalism and Graphic Arts. Never the less, I didn't finish college because I had some conflicts of interest in dealing with the administration not honoring my medical withdrawal. Although I was successful at one thing, that is so very important in my life. I met my husband there."

"My husband who 5 years later gave me a baby girl, a baby girl who does not have Sickle Cell but does have the trait. A Baby Girl who has so much promise that it's a little frightening. My husband and I have banked our daughters cord blood, with the hope that sometime in the not too distant future, will give me New Life!!! I am in the process of deciding when to get the 'Mini Stem Cell Transplant'. I will continue doing what the Lord's will in my life is. I asked Him for the coping skills, to deal with whatever comes my way with SCD, and He gave them to me. I asked Him for a child, when He knew that the child would be healthy and the father would be there, and He did. Now I ask that I get this transplant when He knows that it will be a safe and successful procedure and I know that He will.

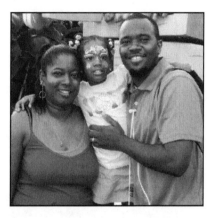

Bridgett, Adaran & Narada Willkie

Well, that's my life in a nut-shell. I know what my purpose in life is now. I am starting a SCD center here in Central Florida and Hope to reach out to many, many, many others who have SCD and need someone that understand it to be there for them.

Let it Begin With me

The World Health Organization (WHO) estimates that over 300,000 children born each year are affected by sickle cell disease and in Africa, more than half of the children born with the disease do not live up to five years.

Touched by Their Stories   **Dan Moore, Sr.**

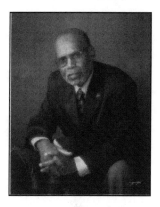

It has been so long ago I don't remember the circumstances under which we met. I do recall she was slender and appeared very fragile. Her name was Telafara. It is the type name you don't easily forget. I do, however, remember our conversation and the first words she said, "I have sickle cell anemia. I am not supposed to be here. I was told I would not live beyond age twelve. I am now 27 and I do not know how long I will last."

Although it was more than 30 years ago, these words are still clear in my mind. Because of my passion to produce films that have some impact, of course my immediate thought was: how can I tell this story and perhaps bring hope to those suffering from this little known illness?

That's when I began my research to learn more about this genetic disease that was peculiar to a segment of our community, primarily Blacks and people from the Mediterranean region.

I soon learned that sickle cell was a very painful condition caused when normal blood cells, which are doughnut shaped, become sickle shaped and block the flow of blood. This causes oxygen, carried by blood cells, not to reach vital organs and can cause irreparable damage.

I was now a lay person with a mission. I had to take on this challenge so that I could help make a difference in the lives of those suffering with the disease and their families who also had to bare a burden.

The questions I had to answer were evident. What is sickle cell disease? When and where did it originate? How is this genetic disorder passed on? What is the life expectancy of those with the disease?

The answers would not come easy. The absence of the internet and quick sources of information made the task more daunting. Yet, I knew there were many suffering from sickle cell and many health professionals working to make a difference.

I began by interviewing doctors working in the field. My first interview was with Dr. Christmas in Philadelphia. I could not forget that name. I often thought to myself, I hope he does not have a daughter and name her Mary. Being called Mary Christmas would certainly be a challenge for any young person. Dr. Christmas referred me to a doctor in Detroit. I flew from my hometown, Philadelphia, Pennsylvania to Detroit to talk to a physician I was told was one of the leading advocates in the field. I don't recall his name but I do remember he talked about the chances of passing on this disorder if both parents have sickle cell trait. He had developed large dice with letters representing the normal gene and the sickle gene. He stated that the chances were one in four that if both parents had the trait that the child would be born with sickle cell.

I set up my camera to film this "rolling of the dice." I was prepared to take as many shots as necessary to capture the roll of the dice that met his predictions. I only had to film one take. As fate would have it, a roll of the dice four times and as predicted, one child was normal, two had the trait and one had the disease.

When I began writing this book, I did not recall the name of the doctor in Detroit. As I began further research I came to a page with a photo of a pioneer in the field of sickle cell. I immediately recognized him as Dr. Charles Whitten. A tall distinguished physician with a most pleasing and warm personality. This came just hours after I began writing this book. The enormous possibilities of the internet, is in some ways incomprehensible. I will address more about Dr. Whitten in the chapter on pioneers.

Now it was up to me to lay this all out on film and hope for wide distribution to help make a difference. Before I could complete the film however, I received a call from a friend of Telafara …she lost her battle and never reached the age of 28.

From there it was off to Accra, Ghana to film what was then the largest hospital on sickle cell in the world. Although we had all of our paper work in order and a letter from the Counsel General of Ghana, it was of little value. Ghana had recently experienced a coup and they were very apprehensive about filming in the country. After many trips to the Embassy, conversations with top officials and several days spent in the hotel just waiting, we finally received word, "the President said, it is O Kay to film." Grabbing our gear and rushing off to the hospital, we set up and took our first shots. Unfortunately, they were also our last shots. Within minutes of setting up, the army officials came with the words, "the President said, you can no longer take pictures."

It was then back to the states to salvage what little I could and begin the arduous task of editing. It was not like today, when you can sit at a computer and move and shift scenes at will. It was the days of film, which meant physically putting film and separate sound tracks on a rack and splicing them together. Then there was sending them to the lab for a two-day process for each effect, dissolve or fade.

The film entitled, *The Doctor Is In*, was finally completed and hopefully served to bring awareness.

Breaking
The Silence

It is estimated that between 70,000 and 80,000 Americans have sickle cell disease, and more than 1,300 babies are born with the condition each year.

Meet Joyce Washington

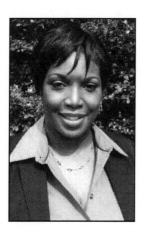

I never imagined the journey my life would have taken with the birth of a child diagnosed with sickle cell disease.

The extent of my knowledge about sickle cell, was that I, and the majority of my family, where trait carriers. I had a cousin that died at the age of 3, and I remember how scared I was that I could die. My mother told me that I could not die because I just carried the trait. I remember asking her what kind did my cousin have that made her die? My mother had to search for an answer and came up with "the kind that can kill you". All I knew was I had the trait, but I never understood what that meant.

As I grew into adulthood, I realized that sickle cell was being referred to by many different names, such as: bad blood, yellow eyes, sickler, and now we call it the silent disease.

I didn't think about it again until just before I got married. My husband- to-be and I went to have a blood test, and they asked if either of us knew if we had the trait. Well, I said, I knew I had the trait, and my fiancée, stated that he

83

did not.   After the birth of my first-born Tayla, the pediatrician told her father and me that she had the sickle cell trait. I seized that moment to ask every question I could about the trait and how one could "catch the disease". The first myth the doctor corrected me on was that you do not catch sickle cell. It is a genetic disorder that you are born with it. The doctor gave me a little 2-sided pamphlet that confused me more. The one good thing I got out of it, was both parents have to carry the trait for a child to be born with the disease. I was consoled with the knowledge that my husband was NOT a carrier and I could NOT have a child that could die with the disease like my cousin.

It was as if life, as I knew it, totally stopped. My heart gripped with fear at the news from the pediatrician that my 3rd daughter Aaron Nicole, was born with sickle cell disease. I did not believe the doctor because I was told that my children could not contract the disease if both parents did not carry the trait, and I believed my husband when he said that he and his family did not carry the trait. His mother even confirmed it at the news that Aaron had the disease. I can only imagine the thoughts that my husband and his family must have had, that I could have been cheating and got pregnant with another man's child, an act I would never do to my family. After my husband was tested, we learned that he was a trait carrier.

The reality of Aaron's diagnosis with sickle cell disease, as I knew it to be "a death sentence," sent me into protective mommy mode. The strength I gained losing my mother to cancer at the age of eighteen kicked me into action. I knew then and there, I was not going to lose my child to this disease.

Saving my daughter's life was my motivation and I read everything I could about the disease and a cure, which wasn't much. I researched the best medical doctors and facilities that specialized in sickle cell. Here in Atlanta, Georgia, Children Aflac Cancer and Blood Disorders Clinics was one of the best in the country. Our long and painful journey began there.

We connected to a very small sickle cell community of which, I noticed, did not have many support services and financial aid to families dealing with sickle cell disease. Being a part of such a small community, I never knew how many people around the world suffered with sickle cell especially adults who suffer. Before I found out how to surf the World Wide Web, I thought the sickle cell life expectancy did not reach in to adulthood. That just showed how ignorant I was in knowing about SC. It saddens me that there was no known cure and that research was underfunded at that time. It was my goal to put Aaron on the path to becoming the longest living sickle cell survivor. I was desperate not to lose my beautiful baby to this disease.

I read about bone marrow/stem cell transplant for sickle cell and discussed it as a possible cure for Aaron.

During the long days and nights, prayers for Aaron flowed. I also began to pray for my sickle cell community at large. I began asking why the sickle cell community lacks in support, awareness, and education. Why was there such a lack of financial support for research to find a cure for all who suffer with SCD? Why are African Americans still, one hundred years after the discovery of SCD here in this country, having such a problem supporting and participating in trial studies and blood and marrow drives?

After researching to find the answer to such questions, a new passion and drive filled my heart that ignited my new mission, - to aid in bringing about a greater awareness and to educate the world at large about sickle cell. With the support of a few people and another mother with children with sickle cell, my co-founder, Ms. Suzanne Gordan, the **F**amily **A**dvocacy **C**oalition for the **E**mpowerment of the Sickle Cell Community, F.A.C.E Foundation, Inc., was born.

FACE Foundation's awareness and cause campaigns will be developed to reduce the lack of knowledge and stigma frequently associated with this chronic generic disease, by disseminating positive images and information about the disorder. Without this effort, those who suffer with Sickle Cell Disease are left with the 100-year-old social stigma of "bad blood" and other negative and embarrassing images.

www.facefoundationinc.org

Meet Aaron Washington

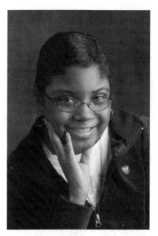

Aaron had severe sickle cell disease. By age 11, she had endured Acute Chest Syndrome, 3 strokes with therapy for recovery, chronic blood transfusions every 3 to 4 weeks, treatment for iron overload, meningitis, countless hospitalizations and doctors and clinic visits.

After she experienced her second stroke while on transfusions, which was needed to prevent her from having strokes, the doctors could not assure her family that the transfusion therapy could prevent Aaron from having life threatening and debilitating strokes that may lead to her death.

"At that point the doctors told her parents about BMT (Bone Marrow Transplant) for sickle cell patients. A perfect sibling match would be the protocol for consideration. They were all tested for a perfect HLA typing, her 2 sisters Tayla and Maya, her brother, Jeremiah, and her father and mother. The tests all came back, NO MATCH! Her family prayed that God would make a way.

During one of Aaron's routine blood transfusions and check-ups, her doctors asked if they would volunteer to consider participating in a research study for severe sickle cell. The study was to try a new treatment for sickle cell using bone marrow transplantation from a close non-matched sibling. The family was told that in order for a successful BMT treatment for Sickle cell the donor and host had to be a 6 out of 6 perfect match. Aaron and her oldest sister, Tayla were a 5 out of 6 match, closes enough to be part of the study. Prayers answered! Hope at last!

Aaron was told about the risks and it would not be easy. They told her about the side effects from the chemo and that it would kill her bone marrow in order to replace it with her sister's. She was told how it would make her sick and how all her long beautiful hair would fall out and how she could develop GVHD (Graft Versus Host Disease) and maybe even rejection. The worse case would be that she could die. Aaron thought a little about it, and said, "I have been in pain all my life, and lots of needles, going back and forth to the hospital, feeling sick all the time, and about my hair, it will grow back. I have no hope with sickle cell, but with God and this BMT I may have a chance." Then, she turned to her mother and said, "Mommy I want to do it." Her mother replied, "O Kay" and went on to say "we never looked back."

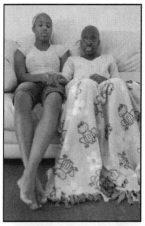

Aaron and sister, Tayla

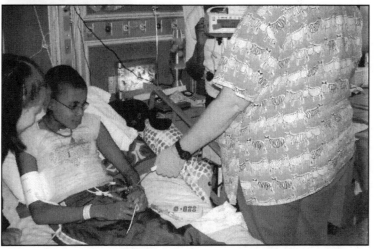

Sunday March 23rd, 2007 check in day at Children's Hospital at Egleston.

Aaron and her family went in with hope, faith and trust in God! Aaron just shined with hope in her heart. She went into surgery to have her central line put in and her own marrow harvested.

Her big sister Tayla checked in on April 3rd for her marrow harvesting to give to her sister. Tayla did not think twice about what she was giving up. She said she would do anything to make her baby sister well. Tayla does not see her gift as a sacrifice. To her, it was something she had to do.

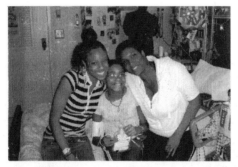 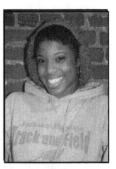

Tayla, Aaron and her mother Joyce   Tayla

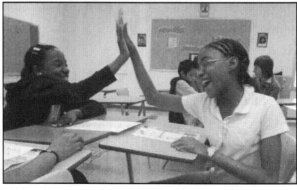

The Surgery was successful, and Aaron is now sickle cell FREE.

Meet Chris Lundy

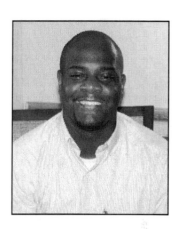

Chris was diagnosed with sickle cell disease when he was two months old after being misdiagnosed earlier. His parents didn't know much about sickle cell, but they knew it was serious enough to take him to Atlanta from their home in Rome, Georgia, where he could be treated. For the next several years Chris had several crises. This would happen about once a year, which pales in comparison to others with the disease. By the time he reached 9th grade, it became more serious and the crises more frequent.

Chris is now twenty two years old and a Student Services Specialist at Georgia Highlands College. He reflects on those days as though it was yesterday. "I remember very vividly", he recalls, "being in and out of the hospital and having several operations. I had my spleen removed when I was two, and had gall bladder surgery at the age of five- it wasn't easy. By the fall of 1999, while in the 10th grade things began to get worse."

"The doctors suggested a marrow transplant. I was nervous about the idea. Having been through surgery before, I knew it would set me back in school and I would have to leave my friends in Rome, Georgia and travel to Atlanta for the treatment. But we have a very close and supportive family and I knew that they were with me. My family planned several donor drives and the doctors at Children's Health Care of Atlanta (CHOA) suggested we test my younger brother who was ten years old. The test would have to be a six point match for the marrow transplant to work. My brother was a perfect six."

Chris' brother, Warren, would then be called upon to possibly save his brother's life. Warren recalls his reaction, "I was really for it. There was no hesitation. It's my brother. Let's get on with it. We have a strong family and we always stick together. I don't like hospitals so my thought was let me get in, get this done, and get out of there. We went in about 6 am and by 2 PM it was all over and they wanted me to stay overnight. My thought was, no, let me get out of here and go home. I was ready to go. I did my part. We left and headed home."

For Chris it was a tremendous blessing and he says he is forever grateful to his brother for saving his life. He also expresses his gratitude to Children's Health Care of Atlanta for the service they provided. Chris states with deep emotion, "The doctors at CHOA were always very concerned and cautious during the entire time. They did not take any short cuts. After surgery I had a brief battle with Graff Versus Host Disease (GVHD) but it was only a temporary setback. I was on mediation from 7 am to 1 pm and then again from 7 pm to 1am."

"On January 17, 2001, I recall as though it was yesterday, I had an experience I will never forget. I was at a basketball game and felt my head itching. I went to scratch my head and then could not take my arm down. I fell forward, face down, on a concrete pavement. I ended up in Egleston Children's Hospital. I have not had any problems since that day."

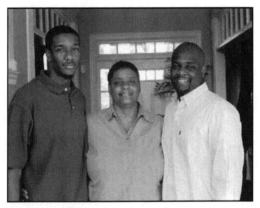

Warren, (mother), Deborah and Chris Lundy

Warren, who is now much taller than his brother Chris, says he would do it all over again if needed. "I only have one brother and I am grateful and humble about what I did. I needed a brother to look up to and go to for advice. I have that brother."

Meet Nile Price

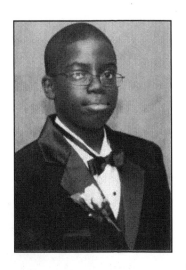

Mrs. Deborah Price gave birth to triplets, Jordan, Nile, and Immanuel. The joy and excitement of giving birth was soon replaced with tears and fear when she received a phone call from the Maryland Health Department telling her that Nile was diagnosed with sickle cell disease.

At exactly thirteen months old Nile had his first pain crisis. He experienced hand-foot syndrome which caused his hands and feet to swell badly. This began the first of many long hospital admissions.

By age five, Nile had already had about 60 to 100 hospital admissions. He had suffered many painful crises, bone necrosis and pneumonias. His family did all they knew to make sure he had as normal a life as his brothers. He played sports but with limitations. He had lots of limitations on his life for more than 13 years.

Nile was taken out of school because he was just too sick to return, and soon after was actually living in the hospital. His hematologist said that he needed a bone marrow transplant because his condition was really getting worse - she feared he would suffer a stroke or other organ damage, all of which is not reversible. The family agreed, but with many reservations and lots of fear.

Nile's two brothers were tested to see if they were a donor match. The family was hopeful and the boys were excited to possibly be a match for their brother. The idea of Nile being cured of this dreadful disease was the best news the family had received in a very long time. The transplant coordinator called two weeks later to say the brothers were not a match. This was a devastating blow, because parents are rarely a match, and Nile's parents weren't. The coordinator said the search would now go to the National Bone Marrow Registry. She informed the family that it could take awhile because of the low number of African Americans on the registry. As the search began, the Price family began to do their part to educate and get people registered. Their son, along with thousands of others, was in need of a lifesaving transplant. The Price family and friends began to organize drives. Nile's mother Deborah states, "Sadly to say, at each drive the turnout to register was incredible, but they all consisted of other races readily agreeing to register to possibly be of help to save my son's life. The drive that was the greatest disappointment was the weekend that the Pittsburgh Steelers were in town for a charity event. Our friends were there to do a drive and there were so many people. We had over eighty people to register that day. The disappointment was the fact that only four of those people were African American. Only two football players registered, even though my child was there talking to countless people. Hundreds of people were there to see the child who was in desperate need of this life saving transplant, and only the people of other races were moved with enough compassion to help. While grateful as we were for them joining the registry, unfortunately they would not be a good match for Nile. We needed an African American donor and we needed one soon."

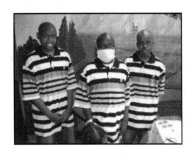

Jordan, Nile, Immanuel

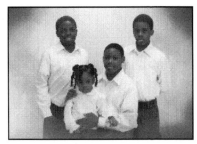

Nile, Olivia, Jordan, Immanuel

Nile and his family thank God for answering prayers. The Bone Marrow Transplant (BMT) Coordinator called with great news. From the National Registry, two perfectly matched donors had been found. While being a matched donor you still have the opportunity to say no, but thankfully the donors were in agreement. The first donor was tested and she agreed to continue with the donation of her bone marrow. On July 21st Nile received his new stem cells, and by the end of August he was 100% donor cells and Sickle Cell Disease free.

Deborah tearfully testifies, "If it had not been for this wonderful woman, my son would still be battling this horrific disease, and I would still be wondering if I'll get to see him graduate from college or get married. Today, thanks to a donor, we are planning his future and enjoying hearing him talk about his plans for becoming a Senator. We did not request to take this journey, but since we had to go through this, I thank God for the person who decided one day to give the gift of life to another person. Our prayer is that other African Americans would give the gift of life by becoming a registered bone marrow donor before it is too late."

"And we know that all things work together for good to them that love God, and to them who are the called according to His purpose." – Romans 8:28

Meet Taylor John - fifteen year old high school student.

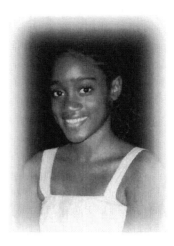

"I'm in 11th grade, and when I grow up I want to be a hematologist. My favorite subject is science. I got an A in science and I will graduate in 2012. I'm going to college. I want to go to Emory, to be a hematologist. I got my mind made up."

Taylor expresses herself so eloquently stating, "I feel thankful that so many people would love to help me, and I'm hoping for one of those people to be a match to save my life - and not just my life but many others. Just because I'm the only face that you see, doesn't mean that I'm the only person that you're helping. You can be a match for any other person out there. You're just signing up with me but you don't have to be my match. That's what I love about this, - it's not just about me. It's about everyone."

"I'll be 16 on my birthday, August 15th. I like dancing. I used to dance with my church, but then my illness came back, so I haven't danced in a while. I like going to sickle cell camp. That is something I really do enjoy. I like spending time with my family down in Florida, and I just like hanging out sometimes going to see movies and being a normal teenager. "

"Really I don't go a lot of places, I mostly stay at home but when I do go out I either go to the mall or go see a movie with my family. My favorite singing group is Mary Mary. I like the song 'God In Me.'"

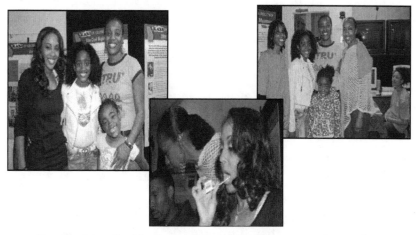

Donor drive for Taylor at The APEX Museum where the JamPoet swabs to join the registry.

Taylor has been on the registry for five years. We pray that she will soon find a match.

Meet Laquontics Gekia Gibson (Kia)

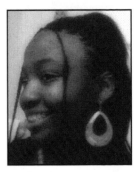

Laquontics Gekia Gibson, (Kia) was born in December, 1993. I was proud to bring her into this world. When they told me I was having a girl I screamed so loud everyone heard me in the waiting room. I always wanted a girl.

Well my story began 10 days after she was born when the doctor told me she had a disease and asked if I knew what sickle cell was. I said yes then they told me everything bad and good. I cried for days. I thought the girl I wanted and got will leave this world at an early age.

We call her Kia. She has gone to the hospital every month for a year staying in a week at a time. She cried at night I never knew what was wrong with her. Her hands would get so big like you could pop them with a pin. We were so scared to touch her but my little baby girl got so much attention. When she was 6 months old she had tubes put in her ears. That was a rough 3 months. When she turned 5 years old every time she ate she would cry about hour later and we didn't know what was wrong. Finally, they took X-rays and found stones in her gall bladder. To the doctor's amazement, she had the surgery and got up and walked the same day. That was a rough 3 months

That same winter she went into the hospital with acute chest syndrome. She had no signs of being sick until one day she ran a high fever at school and the teacher called me to come and pick her up. Her temperature was 104. I rushed her to the doctor and they ran a series of tests. After the tests came back negative, they did a chest X-ray and there it was in both her lungs. She was rushed to ICU and that gave me a scare. I thought this time I am going to lose my child. She stayed there for a month in half and the first night the doctor didn't tell me they did not expect her to live. They decided to put her in a light coma. Then they slowly drained the fluid out off her lungs for 2 weeks. That's the worst thing to see your child asleep, can't talk, can't play- just lay there.

That stay in the hospital was hard on my family but friends and family would come and let me get some sleep in the waiting room. I tried but I couldn't leave my baby girl. Then the day came when the doctor told me they were going to wake her up. I was so happy. She would finally get to open her eyes all the way and talk and see me, even though she felt me there for when I touched her she would squeeze my hand. When we finally got home it was joy. Her brothers were so glad to see her. Then my husband told me I was bankrupt again. I lost my car and house the second time and yet, it did not matter. The most important thing to me was the fact that I still had my baby girl with me.

For the next three years she was not hospitalized as much. While that was great, but the coma left her impaired and adversely affected her school work. She had to go to summer school every year just to keep up. When Kia turned nine I got divorce and moved to Columbia County. They were a lot of help to her and she started to feel good but still stayed back ever year. Most birthdays and holidays were spent in the hospital. Kia is now 15 and has pain in her foot. Every month I'm running to the doctor to see what's wrong. They did not find anything wrong. I then got a second opinion and they found that her blood vessels were deteriorating and they give her aspirin to take for a month. She still has pain. She wants to be a cheer leader so bad but she never gets picked. She tries out every year and she gets angry when she doesn't make it. She tried out for track, basketball, and softball but with the pain she couldn't handle it. I'm proud she tried although she has a brother, Jay, who is a track star and has a lot of medals trophies and she wants to be in the spot light. As a mother who loves her daughter I will continue to seek answers and pray that God will bring us through this.

Meet J. R. Perry

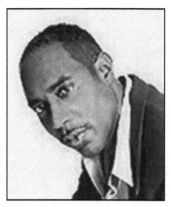

"My son, Jameel Raeshaun Perry was born July 27 1999. Two days after his birth, the doctor said my son, Jameel, had sickle cell anemia, SS TYPE. That was the day my life changed. Jameel's biological mother was very unstable couldn't handle a child with Sickle Cell so 6 days after his birth I had my son as a single father. I was scared and very concerned about my new born son. I began to read everything I could find on sickle cell. I learned how painful sickle cell was an all that Jameel would be facing. So Jameel and I moved from California to Detroit Michigan where he could get the best care."

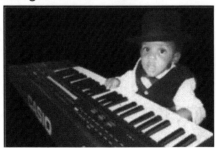

Jameel Raeshaun Perry

"My life changed. I walked away from a smash Talk Show Called the J R Perry Show, my record label, Pro -Per Records AND ALL MY BUSINESS Dealings to be a Sickle Cell Activist -- to help find a Cure- to help educate parents and people in general about sickle cell -to be a voice because I didn't hear any out there. I saw no PSA's on Sickle Cell so I felt it was my duty to be the voice for sickle cell, to fight whatever battle - to open sleeping eyes - to reach out to all so called LEADERS to see why they never talk about sickle cell. I wanted to learn the true history about sickle cell not the watered down version of America's."

"I was seeking the true history. I prayed to get my son a cure. That was my focus and has been since my son was born with sickle cell anemia."

J.R. has indeed dedicated his life to his son. He speaks of how he was even careful while dating to make sure that no one brought any possible infection into his home that could compromise his son's delicate immune system.

J.R. is creator of the worldwide Cure Every Cell Music Tour 2010. It is a concert series to benefit the Sickle Cell Cure Foundation's (SCCF) five year fundraising plan. SCCF is a Oklahoma based nonprofit, 501 (c) (3) organization.

"Let the Truth Be Told"

Meet Sekqueen Carlton-Carew

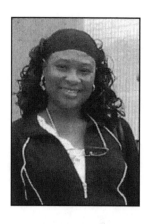

"I am the founder of Coulson sickle Cell foundation. CSCF was one of my dream projects that I wanted to fulfill. I initially wanted to start a children's Home in Sierra Leone in 1996, but did not follow through, due to the civil unrest in Sierra Leone. Little did I know that I would have a Son with special needs, and then finally reality hit me that this might be my calling."

"I was preparing to visit Sierra Leone in 2003 with my son, Sonnie, who has *Sickle Cell SS*. Upon consultation with my son's physicians, I was surprised to learn of the restrictions to which I must adhere to prevent my son from having a "crisis" which is frequent with this disease. Because of the dearth of public medical facilities in Sierra Leone, and the absence of any facility to treat an individual with sickle cell disease at the minimum, specifically one in a crisis, I realized I was taking my son to my homeland at much personal risk. As a mother, the restrictions were necessary for a successful visit, but as a Sierra Leonean, it was unacceptable to know I cannot spontaneously visit home with my son without bringing a variety of medical supplies in anticipation of a crisis."

"It was then I realized there are likely thousands of children with the disease at home; including Sierra Leoneans with children abroad who would like to visit the country but could not do so without the proper medical facilities and professionals, in Sierra Leone."

"At one month old, Sonnie had his first crisis. Since then he has had so any hospitalizations and emergency visits I have lost count. I remember one day, a simple bicycle ride, ended him in the hospital. He had a muscle spasm, and was in so much pain, it turned into a crisis, and he was admitted. His pain was so severe he needed assistance just to walk. His hemoglobin dropped, he required a blood transfusion and ended up staying two weeks in the Hospital missing school and his friends."

"Children with sickle cell disease may sometimes look healthy, but sickle cell disease is unpredictable and can cause pain and damage to the body at any time. He misses a lot of school due to his illness. I remember in one year, he was admitted to the hospital ten times. He is sometimes in and out of the emergency room because of acute chest or infection. Currently, he gets blood transfusion every 4 weeks, due to abnormal TCD (Transcranial Doppler) the blood transfusion helps him to feel better and stay healthy. He is now on a new break through medication (Exjade) that helps with his Iron overload due to frequent blood transfusion."

"My aim is to create awareness, so in the future it can prevent sudden death from infections and crisis in early childhood, and to understand the risk and benefits by educating families about the disease, and helping children to grow into adulthood and live productive lives."

www.coulsonsicklecell.org

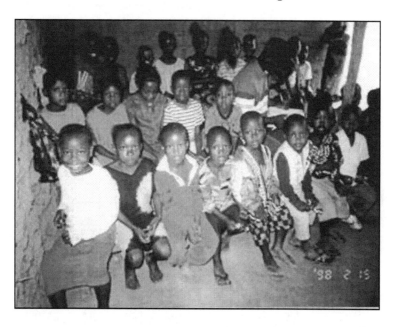

My children in Sierra Leone

Meet Sonnie Coulson John

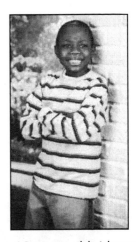

"My name is Sonnie Coulson John. I am 10 years old. I have sickle cell anemia commonly known as Sickle Cell Disease (SCD). I hate to use the word *disease*, because It is not contagious, it is an inherited blood disorder, which causes pain. It affects the red blood cells called hemoglobin in my body. You can only get sickle cell disease by receiving two sickle cell genes, one from each parent who carries a sickle cell gene."

"Sometimes I do get crisis. The logo on this website shows my swollen hand at age one month old. I cannot remember because I was only a month old, but my parents told me that I cried a lot, because it causes me to have pain. I sometimes get sick at home and at school. I miss a lot of days from school due to my illness; in many cases, when I am in crisis, I end up at the emergency room or admitted to the hospital. Now I understand my problems when I am having a crisis."

"I get blood transfusion every four weeks, to help me feel better and stay healthy. When I get sick, I get tired and sleepy. I want to tell other children with sickle cell to drink plenty of water, juices, and no sodas or coffee. We (sickle cell patients) get dehydrated very quickly. Always carry a water bottle and drink plenty of water and always take frequent breaks or rest. Not drinking fluids can help damage our organs in our body. We have to avoid too much heat and cold weather, because that makes us dehydrate and our blood does not flow properly."

"I am on a new breakthrough medication now. Thanks to medical research. It helps me stay healthy. I would like to have other sickle cell children to be my friends and write to me about their experiences with the illness. Please send me an e-Mail to sonniecj@coulsonsicklecell.org. "

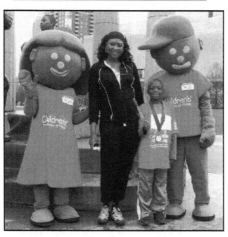

Me and my mother at Children's
Health Care of Atlanta (CHOA)

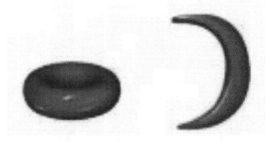

A normal cell and a sickle cell

Sickle Cell Pioneers

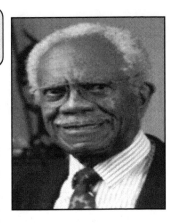

Dr. Whitten formed the Sickle Cell Detection and Information Center,the most comprehensive community program in the country, and facilitated the creation of the National Association for Sickle Cell Disease.

He was best known for his pioneering work in sickle cell anemia screening and development of novel educational tools for teaching children and families with sickle cell anemia. His forceful advocacy paved the way for the routine newborn screening for sickle cell anemia in Michigan and later in the United States.

Dr. Whitten's lobbying efforts on behalf of children with sickle cell anemia also helped push the National Heart Lung and Blood Institute to set up the comprehensive sickle cell center program. A pivotal contribution in toxicology was Dr. Whitten's work at Children's Hospital of Michigan on acute iron poisoning and strategies for its treatment, which developed the standard of care to date. Whitten became program director for the Comprehensive Sickle Cell Center at Wayne State University in 1973.

www.thehistorymakers.com/biography

Daniel Kim Shapiro, PhD

"I am a Biophysicist. My main goal *is to use* light (including polarized light) to learn about biological structure and function.

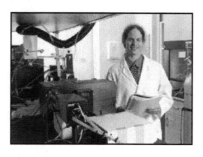

Current interest: Study the effects of Nitric Oxide and Aggregation in biological systems, especially as it relates to diseases such as Sickle Cell Disease."

Kim-Shapiro's pioneering research on sickle-cell anemia and other cardiovascular disorders is well known. He has received several grants from the National Institutes of Health to support his research. His research focuses on nitric oxide, a signaling molecule that is important in maintaining adequate blood flow, regulating blood clotting and other physiological functions. Nitric oxide dysfunction contributes to many diseases including sickle-cell disease, pulmonary hypertension, malaria and stroke.

He is Associate Professor of the Department of Physics at Wake Forest University.

113

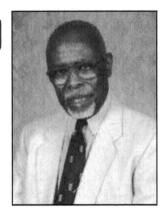

Dr Felix Konotey-Ahulu is one of Ghana's leading scientists (now living in the UK), and one of the world's leading experts in sickle-cell anemia. He has lectured all around the world, and is the author of a major 643-page text, *The Sickle Cell Disease Patient.*

Dr. Konotey-Ahulu is world renown and he was one of the recipients of the Dr Martin Luther King Jr. Foundation Award 'for outstanding research in Sickle Cell Anemia'. In 2004 he was voted among 'The One Hundred Greatest Africans of All Time'.

Between 1965 and 2005 he published more than 200 articles, letters, editorials, book reviews, and comments. Dr Konotey-Ahulu traced the Sickle Cell Gene in his ancestry, with patients' names, generation by generation back to AD 1670, aided by the fact that the hereditary rheumatic syndrome was known to African tribes by specific onomatopoeic names (*hemkom, chwechweechwe, nwiiwii, ahotutuo, nuidudui*) for centuries before it was first described in the USA in 1910. This exercise in genetic genealogy, rare in Medical Archives, helped him develop a discipline of genetic epidemiology to show how polygamy in his forebears produced gene combinations with variations in phenotypic expression of the hereditary syndrome. His invention of the Male Procreative Superiority Index (MPSI), which shed new light on African Anthropogenetics, is the result of this personalized genetic epidemiology.

But the most pertinent qualification of Dr Konotey-Ahulu is that he was born into a Sickle Cell Disease family. He saw siblings in painful crisis even before Linus Pauling in 1949 discovered that an abnormal hemoglobin (S) was the molecular cause of the problem. This fact of having lived with the patients who had hereditary rheumatism as far back as 6 decades ago, and seeing complications like priapism at the tribal setting even before it was described in textbooks has perpetually colored the way Dr. Konotey-Ahulu looks at people with the condition. He has traced the hereditary affliction in his forbears generation by generation to as far back as AD 1670. Dr. Konotey-Ahulu has recently developed a method for writing African Tonal Languages which he has explained in a book titled *Mother Tongue*

www.sicklecell.md

115

The Origin

The Origin

Sickle cell disease has been known to the peoples of Africa for hundreds of years. In West Africa, various ethnic groups gave the condition different names:

- Ga tribe: CHwechweechwe
- Faute tribe: Nwiiwii
- Ewe tribe: Nuidudui
- Twi tribe: Ahotutuo

The repeated syllables are said to mimic the cries of the children suffering from the disease.

- A history of the condition tracked reports back to 1670 in one Ghanaian family.
- In the US in 1846, a paper entitled "Case of Absence of the Spleen" (from the *Southern Journal of Medical Pharmacology*), was probably the first to describe sickle cell disease. It discussed the case of a runaway slave who had been executed. His body was autopsied and found to have "the strange phenomenon of a man having lived without a spleen." Although the slave's condition was typical, the doctor had no way of knowing this as the disease had not yet been "discovered."
- The African medical literature reported this condition in the 1870s, where it was known locally as **ogbanjes** ("children who come and go") because of the very high infant mortality rate caused by this condition.

- The first formal report of sickle cell disease came out of Chicago about 50 years later, in 1910, when a patient of his from the West Indies had an anemia characterized by unusual red cells that were "sickle" shaped.
- In 1922, after three more cases were reported, the disease was named "sickle cell anemia.
- In 1948, using the new technique of protein electrophoresis, Linus Pauling and Harvey Itano showed that the hemoglobin from patients with sickle cell disease is different than that of others. This made sickle cell disease the first disorder in which an abnormality in a protein was known to be at fault.

What is Sickle Cell Disease?
- It is a group of inherited red blood cell disorders.
- It is the most common genetic disease in the US.
- *Normal red blood cells are round like doughnuts and they move through small blood tubes in the body to deliver oxygen. Sickle red blood cells become hard, sticky and shaped like sickles used to cut wheat. When these hard and pointed red cells go through the small blood tubes, they clog the flow and break apart. This can cause pain, damage and a low blood count or anemia.*

What makes the red cell sickle?

- There is a substance in the red cell called hemoglobin that carries oxygen inside the cell. One little change in this substance causes the hemoglobin to form long rods in the red cell when it gives away oxygen. These rigid rods change the red cell into a sickle shape.

How do you get Sickle Cell?

- You inherit the abnormal hemoglobin from both parents who may be carriers of the sickle cell trait or parents with sickle cell disease.
- About 2.5 million African-Americans (1 in 12) are carriers (AS) of the sickle cell trait. People who are carriers may not even be aware that they are carrying the S allele!

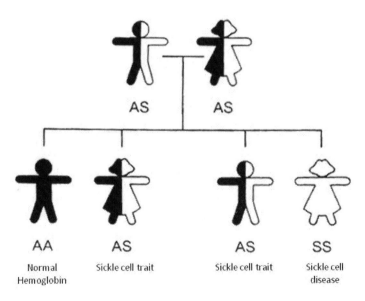

If both parents have the sickle cell trait (S), the chances are one in four that the child may be born with sickle cell disease.

The Challenge

The Challenge
By The JamPoet

If I can give a portion of my life, yet still live to see the gift
I'd lift my hands and volunteer
I'd agree freely the opportunity to free me
Of my tears for the years
I've felt the families
Fear of losing their loved one
I'd mine my marrow like diamonds
A priceless miracle
I'd lay my reservations down at the feet of odds
Because I live by the grace of faith in my higher power
I am empowered to change someone's final hour
To infinite minutes of precious seconds of second chances
I have the power to stand on the summit of someone's
circumstances
And make heroic advances towards the reward of saving a life
I absorb all my lessons
And countless soul searching sessions
And proceed to act kindly
Taking every good deed in me
And unselfishly giving
A harvest of going against the grain
There's no pain id feel that would match
Someone's journey through this life altering disease
There's no pain id feel that would match
The many heart wrenching pleas
Families make time after time
In order to find and remind the races
That they are racing to spare a beloveds life
My sigh is a sign of last breaths and stolen moments
The pain and stress in ones chest
When endure is all they got left

We forget
Of all things out of our control
This isn't it
Each one that is eligible holds a miracle
In order to move you just need one
One daughter, one mother, one sister, one brother,
One loved one, husband, or wife
It's one deed, one match, one victory for life
What's painfully true is many will draw
Their last breath waiting on you
From this day forward I pay forward
The love for my community with my name on a registry
Too many times I think what if it were me
Too many times I didn't want to believe
There is a miracle waiting on me
My weight in miracle gold is me
I hold the key to life
The shortlist it's not long
The waiting list doesn't have long
The greatest gift you can give
Is affording someone a chance to live
They say all the world's a stage
And a hand extended to one in need
Is a hand that has been well played
When you are called to act
Are you moved or dissuade?
When it comes to Marrow for Life
Will you play it safe or will you save?
Register Today

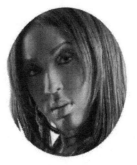

The JamPoet

Produced by Marrow for Life, Inc.
135 Auburn Ave. Atlanta, GA 30303
In collaboration with
FACE Foundation, Inc. & SCD Soldier Network, Inc.

Made in the USA
Charleston, SC
15 August 2011